KETO FOR LIFE

28 Day Fat-Fueled Approach To Weight Loss

Barbara Miller

"In my forties after gradually gaining weight and finally deciding to do something about it, I discovered to my dismay that my old tried-and-true weight loss methods no longer worked. After some research, I decided to try a Keto diet, but the learning curve was steep. I would stare hungrily into my refrigerator and pantry baffled by what I could eat. Then, a friend handed me this book and it all became SO EASY! This brilliant guide tells you what to eat and how to stack meals. I was thrilled when I easily lost 25 pounds in 4 months!!"

— Joleen Firek, MI

KETO FOR LIFE

28 Day Fat-Fueled Approach To Weight Loss

Barbara Miller

"A wise man ought to realize that health is his most valuable possession."

— Hippocrates

OTHER BOOKS WRITTEN BY BARBARA

How to Write a Book and Tell Your Story

Easy Steps to Write, Publish, and Promote Your Book

Dancing in Rhythm with the Universe

10 Steps to Choreographing Your Best Life

Dancing in Rhythm with the Universe Journal

You Lost Your Marriage Not Your Life

How to Create the Life You Want Your Way

Positive Thoughts Journal

You Lost Your Marriage Not Your Life

Disclaimer

The intention of this book is to provide information and encouragement to the reader. It is not intended to counsel or give medical advice in any way. The material in this book is the author's opinion only.

The author is not a doctor and does not treat or diagnose any medical conditions. The information in this book is presented as a result of the author's research and not intended to replace any advice given by your doctor. All the information in this book can be researched and verified by the reader. There are many other resources available regarding information contained in this book. The reader is advised to do their own research on topics herein discussed. The references used do not imply that the companies or individuals endorse this book.

2019 Barbara & Company International, Inc.

Trade Paperback Edition

Published in the United States by Barbara & Company International, Inc.

ISBN: 978-0-9881852-5-8

Library of Congress Control Number:2019912488

Page design & typography by GoMyStory.com/John W Prince

This book in not intended to substitute or replace the advice of your physician, or to replace any treatments prescribed by your doctor. The intention of providing this information is to help you make informed decisions regarding your health. Always consult your doctor before adopting the dietary suggestions in this book.

Printed in the United States of America

Barbara & Company International, Inc.

Barbara@BarbaraAndCompany.com.

Dedication

This book is dedicated to my mother 'Beatrice Marie' who lost her life bravely battling heart disease. You are loved and missed, Momma.

FORWARD

Paul Emberger, Jr

Barbara Miller asked me to write this forward after we spoke at a writers' event, we both attended. She was displaying her book *KETO for LIFE.* The book caught my eye because I recently had become an enthusiastic practitioner of the Ketogenic Diet, not because I was someone who tried all the new diets, but instead, to control my diabetes. She wanted a forward by someone who was successful making the lifestyle change to Keto; that would be me.

In 1992 I was diagnosed with Type 2 Diabetes. My doctor started me on the ADA[1] diet and I started exercising. I stopped eating a lot of my favorite foods, and that was depressing.

With the diet and exercise I was keeping the blood sugar under control. Then for some unknown reason the blood sugar levels went up. I had to begin testing every morning. The doctor started me on Sulfonylureas and soon added Metformin (diabetes medications).

After ten years on the ADA diet I began to have some episodes of hypoglycemia[2]. It was scary! My A1c[3] results were always between 6.0 and 7.3, definitely diabetic.

Fast forward to August 1, 2017 about 7 a.m. My Fasting Blood Glucose result was 223, and I was now Type 2 Diabetic. My fasting blood sugar had been all over the map for the last month, from 69 to 225[4].

My medications had recently been changed from Lantus (long acting insulin) to a new type of diabetic medication, plus another diabetic medication I had been on previously for 20 years.

I had started Lantus the year before and the results were just okay. I still had spikes of high blood sugar and dangerous bouts of low blood sugar.

In May of 2017 I was informed that I had reached the Medicare "donut hole" and that prescriptions were going to cost me a lot more this year. It was depressing!

I was paying a lot of money for medicines that didn't seem to work very well. I could not go anywhere without taking glucose tablets with me. Soon I was suffering from all the secondary disorders brought about by diabetes mellitus.

Additionally, for over 20 years I

suffered from the side effects of Metformin; chronic diarrhea.

There had to be a better way!

Unfortunately, I did not know about Barbara Miller, or her book, which could have saved me a lot of time and misery. I started researching everything I could find about diabetes. I looked in medical books, research studies, history, and nutrition texts.

A single idea kept reappearing. Diabetes is the condition that occurs when your body cannot properly use carbohydrates. That idea was stated in nearly every reference source I read.

Then I had my "Duh" experience. If carbohydrates are associated with the symptoms of diabetes, then DON'T EAT CARBOHYRATES! Barbara reached the same conclusions and she presented them in her book in a clear and logical way.

At this time my blood glucose levels ranged from 71 to 287; from hypoglycemic to hyperglycemic and everywhere in between! I was not in control of my diabetes or my life.

My next discovery was the Ketogenic Diet. Apparently, I was not the only person to make the discovery that diabetes and carbohydrates are related. After reading everything I could find on the Ketogenic Diet, I informed my wife that I wanted to try this new diet.

She said she would work with me and she has ever since. She knew nothing about "Keto," but she dove into the subject and began preparing ketogenic recipes. I decided that this was only going to work if I gave it a 100% effort.

I stopped taking all my diabetic medications except for one Metformin a day. I tested my blood sugar four times a day, and recorded the results. After two weeks I stopped all diabetic medications.

Probably not smart since I had not discussed any of this with my doctor, but I was determined give this ketogenic approach a chance to work.

My wife, Arleen, tried hundreds of recipes. She got better and better at creating great Ketogenic meals. My blood sugars were now below 120 whenever during the day I tested.

I was losing weight as well! In fact, I was also losing my middle-aged spread. The best surprise outcome was my wife was losing weight as well and was keeping it off. And, she was losing dress sizes which made her happy. Her hard work helping me had helped her reach goals she had not been able to achieve with other diets.

In late September 2017 I was due for my semiannual checkup. I gathered all my blood tests and went to my doctor to make my case.

By this point my fasting blood glucose was between 120 and 130 every day. It was higher than I wanted, but more consistent than it had ever been on drugs! I had no episodes of hypoglycemia (seriously low blood sugar). A huge risk had been removed from my life.

I was also afraid that my cholesterol numbers were going to be disastrous with the high fat diet I was consuming to get into ketosis[5]. My wife was similarly fearful for her own cholesterol levels, even though she was, and is, very healthy.

Today, both of us have high HDL (good cholesterol) and low LDL (bad cholesterol) which is what the doctors want. We did not get those test results by avoiding fatty foods. In fact, we ate lots of animal fat, eggs, butter, cheese, and cream, but very few carbohydrates.

In September 2018, not only was my A1c below 7, it was 5.6! My A1c in April 2019 was 5.4, below what is considered pre-diabetic. I never take antacids anymore. I don't eat snacks at night. In fact, I seldom snack at any time.

Today I feel better, I look better, and I have fewer aches and pains. My wife lost four dress sizes. I lost two inches off my waist. My weight today is what it was when I graduated high school. Both our weights have stayed steady for nearly two years now.

By the way, don't worry about the footnotes. They are only there because my part of this book is at the beginning. When you finish the book, you won't need footnotes.

When I realized that ketogenic is a lifestyle, and not a diet, it got easier to do. A key issue for success is knowing what you are actually eating.

Until I started paying attention, I had no idea how many of the foods on grocery shelves have added sugars, flours, and syrups; all carbs!

Once you know what to eat, the Keto Diet takes care of itself. It was tough to give up all those "comfort" foods, but the rewards have been terrific, and the "comfort" was an illusion.

You will see later in Barbara Miller's book how your body responds to carbohydrates, and how they make you feel good while they destroy your metabolism.

Restaurants are more challenging than grocery stores for the ketogenic dieter. In the store you can read the ingredients. In a restaurant, recipes are often secret, or at least not published on the menu. What's in that sauce you had? Was there a lot of bread filler in those crab cakes?

Barbara Miller's book helps to explain what to look for when dining out, and what you can easily make at home. Keto is the way we live today. We are healthier than ever.

Keto for Life by Barbara Miller will help you understand what ketogenesis is. It will also help you to find new ways of eating and preparing food. She explains some important concepts you need to understand to be successful with Keto.

Everything I discovered the hard way about carbohydrates and my health was in her book. Rather than as a guide to my own ketogenesis, it confirmed my research and conclusions; I wasn't crazy.

That made the book a companion that helped me remember that what my wife and I were doing has a scientific basis. It IS NOT A FAD DIET! Diabetes no longer controls my life; I do.

Even if you are not diabetic you will be healthier and feel better when you get the sugar / carbohydrate monkey off your back. Keto is For Life!

Good luck on your journey to better health. The road map to better health is in the pages that follow.

Paul Emberger, Jr

June 4, 2019

---

1 American Diabetes Association

2 Dangerously low blood glucose level.

3 The primary diagnostic test for Type 2 Diabetes

4 American Diabetes Association recommends 80 to 130 for non-diabetics.

5 Ketosis is the process where the body burns fat for energy instead of glucose

Paul Emberger, Jr. earned his BS and MS with a major in Psychology at Towson State University. He was employed as a Professor at Brookdale Community College in Lincroft, NJ, and at Rutgers Graduate School of Education in New Brunswick, NJ as Adjunct Instructor. He switched careers to Information Technology and was employed at Bell Laboratories, Merrill Lynch, J.P. Morgan Chase Bank, and CSX

Paul retired in 2009 and now lives in The Villages, Florida with his wife Arleen.

KETO FOR LIFE

28 Day Fat-Fueled
Approach To Weight Loss

PART 1

INTRODUCTION

“

Ketones are actually the preferred fuel source for the muscles, heart, liver, and brain. These vital organs do not handle carbohydrates very well; in fact, they become damaged when we consume too many carbs.

”

– Eric Westman,[1] author of *Keto Clarity: Your Definitive Guide to the Benefits of a Low-Carb, High-Fat Diet*

“

Ketones are an efficient fuel for human physiology without increasing the production of damaging free radicals. Ketosis allows a person to experience nonfluctuating energy throughout the day as well as enhanced brain function and possibly resistance to malignancy.

– Dr. David Perlmutter,[2] author of *Grain Brain* and *The Brain Maker*

INTRODUCTION

The ugly truth

Are you sick and tired of yo-yo dieting and struggling to stick to a diet that promises to give you awesome results and delicious food to eat? Instead, you eat tasteless microwave food with a list of ingredients you cannot even pronounce.

All the while trying to convince yourself that this will work and you will finally get that weight off, only to be grossly disappointed—again! Oh, you get the weight off alright, only to depressingly watch it creep back on with a vengeance, weighing more after the diet than before.

I can promise you that if you follow what is laid out in this book, you will succeed. How do I know this? Because I have experienced it firsthand. In the past, I have personally tried numerous weight loss plans, and they just do not work!

The very worst one ever was the Cabbage Soup Diet. I was so miserable with the worst stomach ache, and by the end of the third day, I was physically ill.

I have researched nutrition, studied health and wellness for many years, and have read nearly every weight loss book on the market. In my opinion, the ketogenic diet is the best plan I have ever tried, with superior results that affect the entire body. I encourage you to try it for yourself.

One of the biggest challenges of Keto for life is getting your body to a state of burning fat instead of sugar. Some will have a more difficult time than others as we are not all metabolically the same, and have a different level of activity, body fat, and muscle.

What on earth is a ketogenic diet?

Keto is the way you were meant to eat.

In a keto diet, your body uses its body fat for energy. Insulin is your fat storing hormone, but a keto diet forces insulin levels to drop, thus causing your body to burn fat.

You have probably heard the term *ketosis.* ***Ketosis occurs when the body does not have adequate glucose for energy; it will resort to burning stored fat.***

This process called ketosis is set in motion by adopting a ketogenic diet.

We are not talking about consuming artificial fats like artery-clogging partially hydrogenated oils and trans fats. Healthy fats are found in olive oil, coconut oil, avocado oil and avocados, cheese, butter, eggs, meat, and many other natural real foods.

Ketosis is the result of consuming the proper balance of high fat, moderate protein, and controlled low-carb diet.

Both the brain and heart get their energy from ketones when glucose is unavailable. If followed properly, the body will produce ketones as fuel instead of glucose. Carbohydrates get broken down into sugar and deposited as fat.

Once you abandon packaged foods, artificial ingredients, and unhealthy oils, and replace them with real food, you will be shocked at what you have been missing!

There are no counting calories as you begin eating foods like juicy steaks, pork chops, and broccoli drizzled with butter. Your breakfast will give you a reason to jump out of bed: buttery eggs with sausage patties and sautéed spinach.

I will provide several choices to keep you excited and ready to take the last challenge with food you will ever need to get that excess weight off once and for all and keep it off!

It is impossible to lose weight if you continue eating the same carbohydrate dense food you have been consuming. We are going to change that scenario, so keep reading!

If you continue on a low-fat diet, it is almost guaranteed that obsession for food will be your primary thought every day.

The key to success of the keto diet is to move the body away from using sugar as its primary fuel source and towards burning fat.

As the body adapts to burning fat for fuel, it converts fat into ketones, which are then burned for fuel.

Make "Keto for Life, 28 Day Fat-Fueled Approach to Weight Loss," your new lifestyle eating plan. Watch the pounds roll off as you enjoy real amazing food that is not only filling and satiating, but full of satisfying flavor and texture, and it is the RIGHT food!

Don't let the past equal your now. It is not your fault that you have been led down a deadly path by our own government, pharmaceuticals, and health care providers.

I still remember watching my mother stir a packet of yellow dye into our "heart healthy" margarine, which was nothing more than artery-clogging oil. I remember vividly watching her and asking what she was doing. She said, "This is our new butter, the government says we should eat this instead of butter, and it will keep us healthy."

I also recall a family friend stopping by for a visit when I was about nine years old. I never forgot the story he told about how he worked for a food bank; they gave out butter and cheese to those on welfare.

He said the warehouse was stacked to the ceiling with butter and cheese and he thought it was a crime to give these products to those less fortunate when the government instructed the rest of us to eat oil!

He didn't know that they were being supplied with healthy food while the rest of us were being poisoned!

My mother ate margarine most of her adult life until she died of congestive heart failure from chronic heart disease. As many times as I begged her not to eat margarine, her words were still the same, "My doctor said margarine is good for me."

As time went on, many began to see reports coming out about the dangers of trans fats and its link to heart disease.

I know from my own experience several years ago, when I had started gaining weight and had no idea why. I was eating everything that was touted as healthy.

A friend told me he was eating all kinds of pasta every day and was so excited to learn that they were good for him. I decided to try it too.

A year later, he had put on thirty pounds! I gained fifteen pounds before I was shocked into reality. While visiting with my elderly neighbor, out of the blue, she said, "Barbara, I believe you are taking on some weight."

I was stunned and speechless, but the wake-up call was received. I felt like a sinking tugboat. What on earth was wrong?

I had been eating no-fat cardboard cookies, Cheerios, oatmeal, shredded wheat, soy milk, and whole wheat toast. This was supposed to be good for me right? ***Wrong!***

I have always been a researcher and known by my friends and family as a health nut. I learned early on that carbs were not my friend!

Sadly, though, I still did not know what was happening to me at the time or why. I was not eating huge amounts of food. I get this story often from both men and women, and it is always the same, "I cannot seem to lose weight, and I really do not eat that much."

Unfortunately, it does not take a lot of food to gain weight, especially if you are consuming all the wrong foods and in the wrong combinations.

It is now common knowledge that trans fats cause heart disease and interferes with good cholesterol. I was one of the lucky ones, as I did not like margarine and opted for real butter.

Then we moved to a farm when I was ten and had our own butter. In my adult life, whenever I visited my mother, she always bought butter for me. However, she continued to eat her 'heart healthy' margarine.

The fat-free craze was and still is a disaster!

I am shocked at how numerous people sadly believe that eating low fat is the only way to weight loss. They cannot understand why their waist line continues to expand and their weight gain is off the charts.

We are going to be looking closely at the real problem, and then zero in on ways to solve it.

This book will lay out a plan and a path for you to follow to take any guesswork out of your new food regimen.

You will be eating real food and lots of it, allowing you to feel totally satiated.

Kick the yo-yo diets to the curb, along with cardboard cookies, and learn once and for all the very best and most efficient way to get that weight off and more importantly—keep it off!

Weight gain and flat-out obesity are caused by two things, diet and lack of activity.

Yes, I mean exercise.

Sadly, a sedentary lifestyle and the food you eat can lead to obesity, which can lead to type 2 diabetes. According to the American Diabetes Association, "Diabetes is a problem with your body that causes blood glucose (sugar) levels to rise higher than normal. This is also called *hyperglycemia*. Type 2 diabetes is the most common form of diabetes."

They go on to say that your body does not use insulin properly, and when this happens, the result is called *insulin resistance*. The pancreas attempts to make up for it by producing extra insulin, but cannot make enough insulin to keep your blood glucose levels normal.

Once diagnosed with type 2 diabetes, quality of life will suffer. Type 2 diabetes can lead to heart disease, Alzheimer's, kidney failure, blindness, liver disease, loss of limbs, and nerve damage.

My former husband was an Internal Medicine Physician, and occasionally I would go on hospital rounds with him. He was also the medical director of two nursing homes, and this is what really opened my eyes.

The last place you or I want to be is in a nursing home. Several had lost limbs from diabetes, and many suffered the effects of stroke and dementia. Yes, I know there could be other factors involved, but seeing this scenario for myself on several occasions certainly gave me pause for thought on how I treat my amazing body.

On July 17, 2008, *The New England Journal of Medicine* posted results of "Weight Loss with a Low Carbohydrate, Mediterranean, or Low Fat Diet." This two-year study involved 322 participants who were moderately obese. They divided them into three separate groups and assigned each group one of the three mentioned diets. Only the low-carb diet had no restricted calories.

The study surprised mainstream medicine as the low-carb diet showed the most favorable results with the greatest weight loss and reduction in cholesterol and lowered triglycerides.

The Mediterranean diet also had favorable results for diabetic subjects in reducing inflammation and controlling glucagon and insulin levels.

The low-fat came in last!

Dr. Robert Atkins,[2] author of *New Diet Revolution,* would have loved seeing the results of this study. He fought mainstream medicine for years, desperately trying to prove that low-carbohydrate high fat diet was the healthiest way to eat.

I watched him berated for his low-carbohydrate high fat diet by another doctor on a talk show. I wish he could have lived to wallow in the, "I told you so!" This is so amazing! We can finally kick the low-fat fad diets to the curb and enjoy real flavor, fat, and texture without guilt.

In 2015, Dr. David Ludwig[3] of Harvard, along with Dr. Dariush Mazaffarian discussed their findings regarding low-fat diets in the Journal of the American Medical Association. *Dr. Mazaffarian declared:*

"Low-fat diets have had unintended consequences, turning people away from healthy high-fat foods and towards foods rich in added sugars, starches, and refined grains. This has helped fuel the twin epidemics of obesity and diabetes in America. We really need to sing it from the rooftops that the low fat diet concept is dead. There are no health benefits to it."

No, this is not another Atkins Diet, but there are similarities. The Atkins Diet is extremely rigid and not right for everyone.

Even though this diet is low carb and fat friendly, it is far less rigid than Atkins.

However, where we separate company with the Atkins Diet is that we will not be eating high protein, wheat, and grain. Although one important similarity is that we do not count calories—we count carbs!

Dr. Atkins teaches that you will never be able to control your weight until you learn to control carbohydrates! It is so doable and vital for quality of life. Dr. Atkins also states that too much insulin released in the body can be a direct result of consuming too many carbohydrates. In other words, you are not getting fat because you eat too much; you are getting fat because of what you eat!

Low-fat diets are a disaster, and we should avoid them at all costs!

Carbohydrates dominate the government's old Food Guide Pyramid. It promotes eleven servings per day from the whole grains bottom portion! Talk about encouraging obesity.

That is insanity! What a disaster this pyramid has been for our society.

They have now presented what is called My Pyramid in an effort to rein in obesity, but according to the Harvard Department of Nutrition, they simply turned the old pyramid on its side and are promoting the same heavy concentration of carbohydrates, which Harvard says is because of pressure from special interest groups in Washington.

The first triangle in the governments new My Pyramid is grains, and the other larger triangle is dairy. If you eat heavy on grain and heavy on dairy, heavy is what you will be! Although, some dairy is actually healthy for you and I will explain the best choices. Steer away from low-fat, low-calorie, and low-sodium foods as when they are void of fat and flavor, so sugar is added for flavor. ***Don't be fooled!***

The only new recommendation on the new My Pyramid is the stair steps going up the side to promote exercise, which you will definitely need if you follow My Pyramid. Don't buy into their attempt to fool you into believing you can still eat anything you want if you just add exercise. We are going to make our own pyramid, designed to keep you strong, healthy, and enjoying life.

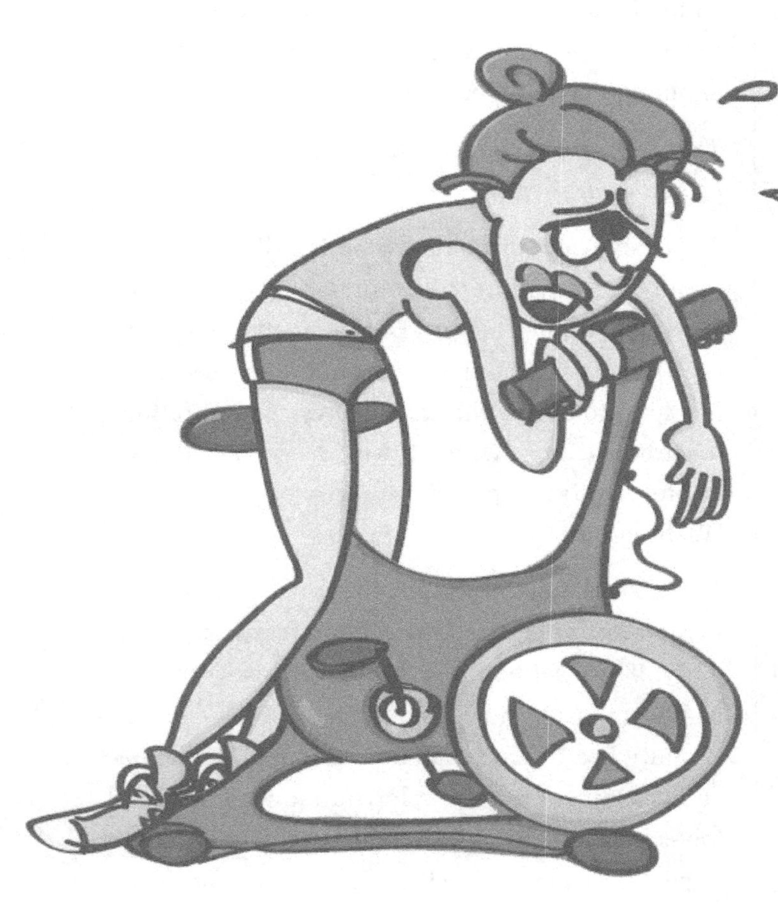

I watch numerous overweight individuals running on treadmills, riding stationary bikes, pumping incredibly heavy weights, dancing and doing various types of exercise.

Unfortunately, no matter how hard they work and how much sweat pours off their brow, they cannot seem to lose the fat. Could it possibly be that they are all in lather for nothing?

After all, if you exercise more and eat less food, shouldn't you be losing weight?

This book is going to answer all your questions and tell you in plain English exactly why this approach does not, never has, and never will work.

CHAPTER ONE

WHAT ON EARTH HAPPENED?

Our family moved to a farm when I was ten. It was a healthy move for us kids. I loved the fruit orchard most of all, and right outside my bedroom window was a cherry tree. I could even reach out the window and grab a few cherries. There were so many new flavors. We spent every spring, summer, and fall working on the neighboring farms picking cucumbers, onions, beans, and potatoes. In the fall, it was wheat harvesting time. The wheat was tall and golden, the perfect picture of "amber waves of grain." Modern wheat is less than half as high as it was thirty to forty years ago. What happened? Enter hybrid wheat. Due to cross-breeding with other stains to create a dwarf plant that produces a high yield of wheat. Due to this tactic, we managed to strip the valuable nutrients right out of the plant.

CHAPTER ONE

"If you don't take care of your body—you won't have any place to live." — Dr. Wayne Dyer

What on Earth Happened?

I went to school in the late fifties and sixties, and like the typical school kid, our lunch consisted of tuna fish, peanut butter, or bologna sandwiches on white Wonder Bread.

The best part was the Hostess Twinkies, Snowballs, or Hostess Cupcakes. They came in twin packs, and we had to split it with a sibling as we were allowed only one single cupcake each.

Our breakfast was Wheaties, cornflakes, Cheerios, shredded wheat or oatmeal. On weekends, we had bacon and eggs with toast or pancakes. We were not a well to do family by any means, and fortunately, we were not allowed to snack between meals, although it did not seem fortunate at the time.

Once school was out, we rushed home which was a two-mile trek and fixed one of the only two things allowed, popcorn or bread. We nearly wore out the toaster, and of course, we popped our popcorn with Crisco oil, but who knew?

Raiding the refrigerator was out of the question as we had strict rules that we might be eating that night's dinner. Not to mention there wasn't much in our refrigerator anyway. Our diet in those days was nutritionally lacking, but it sure followed the original government pyramid!

Dr. William Davis,[3] and his *New York Times* best seller, *Wheat Belly, Lose the Wheat, Lose the Weight, and Find Your Path Back to Health,* exposed the disastrous effects wheat has had on the overall health of our population in the United States as well as many other countries. Dr. Davis is a preventive cardiologist who became increasingly alarmed by men and women who were extremely fat, and some who were considered morbidly obese.

Accommodating 350-pound patients in medical offices, hospitals, and ambulances has become a real problem. We all know about the challenges for airplane passengers and crew when an obese person tries to squeeze into a too-small seat.

On a recent flight, I was amazed as the flight attendants scurried around trying to accommodate an extremely large passenger who was trying to squeeze between two other large passengers.

If you see yourself described here, know that it is not all your fault.

We have been instructed by our own government that in order to be healthy, we must eat more heart healthy whole grains, cereal, pasta, bread, desserts, and to consume fat-free food.

Please believe me when I tell you that this is NOT TRUE! You are not entirely to blame for your weight gain. They are still telling people to eat vegetable oil and wheat. We have all been led down a deadly path, but it does not have to be a dead-end path for you. We can fix this. You deserve to be well and you deserve to be healthy and trim.

Our dinner consisted of some form of meat, mostly fried, along with potatoes, and a vegetable. My dad was not big on salad, calling it rabbit food. This was the standard meal for farmers in those days.

There was always bread if you were still hungry, but no dessert until Sunday, other than the one treat in our lunch during the school year.

Occasionally on Friday night when our mother bought groceries, she would get one small box of candy for us to share: Mounds, Stars, or Non-Pareils. We never had soda pop. On rare occasion we got to have ice cream which was a big hit.

Sunday lunch was special with pot roast, roasted chicken, or ham and, of course, the Sunday dessert.

> *Many of us for a long time have believed the dietary guidelines were pointing in the wrong direction. It is long overdue.*
>
> – Steven Nissen,[6] chairman of the department of cardiovascular medicine at the Cleveland Clinic

> *2015 Dietary Guideline for Americans will no longer include warnings about dietary cholesterol, which for decades has been wrongfully blamed for causing heart disease.*
>
> – Dr. Mercola of mercola.com,[4] a health and wellness website.

The guidelines now state: ***"Cholesterol is not a nutrient of concern for overconsumption."***

Well, it is about time!

Many doctors still prescribe cholesterol lowering drugs to their patients totally ignoring the new evidence. If this is you, do your own research and challenge your doctor!

I am not a doctor, and I am not suggesting that you stop taking your medicine, but you do have the right to question everything you are putting in your amazing body.

The government "My Pyramid" that we talked about earlier shamefully has allotted the largest slice of pie, pun intended, to the wheat section and a tiny sliver section to protein.

This is wrong, and if you continue to follow this disproportionate difference, eating huge amount of grain, namely wheat, and skimping on fat and protein, you are doomed to an unhealthy existence.

The results of this diet will leave you fat, unhealthy, unmotivated, depressed, and possibly stricken with diabetes, heart disease, cancer, celiac disease, irritable bowel syndrome, ulcerated colitis, or Crohn's disease.

Only you can stop this madness and take charge of the only life and the only moments you have. I don't want you to just be alive, I want you to live!

Take back your life. Get mad as hell, get passionate, and above all, get healthy!

The government took such flack about their new pyramid; they were forced to replace it with "My Plate."

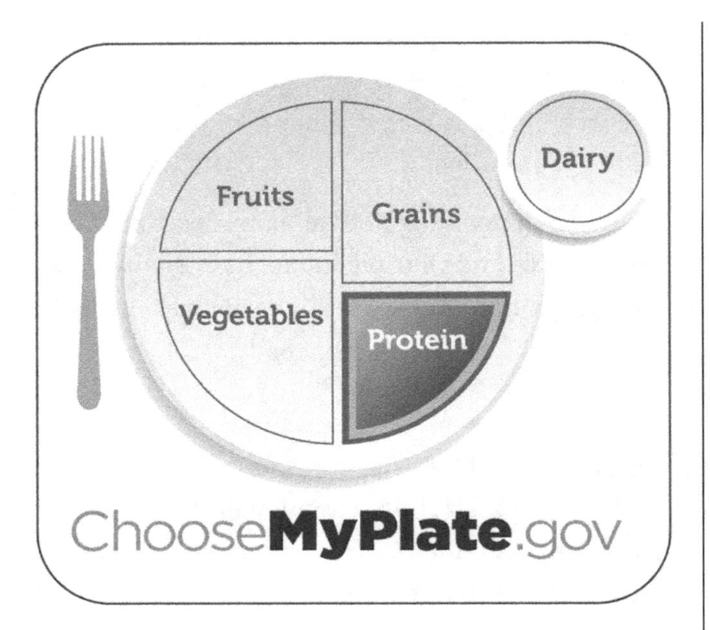

Take a look at the picture of the government's "My Plate" on the left and see that grains are still holding a big piece of the plate, and the portions are way off for a healthy diet.

The US Surgeon General's efforts to help Americans get a handle on obesity is still the 'same ole' advice. Eat low-fat foods and increase whole grains.

This is the very same advice that got us into this disastrous mess in the first place!

The more your waist begins to expand, the risk of developing Type II diabetes grows exponentially right along with it.

The cost of treating diabetes has now surpassed cancer cost. This surge is directly correlated with excess wheat and sugar consumption.

We now have a nation of overweight, wheat, and sugar stuffed, insulin resistant diabetics!

As more carbohydrates are consumed, the pancreas releases more insulin. This constant onslaught to the pancreas damages its ability to stabilize insulin, and blood glucose levels rise.

As visceral fat increases, so does the threat of diabetes.

Dr. Mark Hyman, author of *Eat Fat, Get Thin: Why the Fat We Eat Is the Key to Sustained Weight Loss and Vibrant Health*, states that in 1960, only 1 in 100 people in the U.S. had type 2 diabetes. However, now a shocking 1 in 10 have type 2 diabetes!

Dr. Hyman also states that since the 1980s, type 2 diabetes rates have increased to 700 percent, with 1 in 3 Americans now considered obese. Sadly, those numbers are predicted to increase, not only with adults, but children and teenagers as well!

This book will reveal what is going on and how to get a handle on this tragic growing epidemic.

Dr. Mercola, a well-known health advocate, posted an article on October 28, 2013, regarding the 10 sources of calories in the American diet.

Number one is grain based desserts, number two is yeast breads, number three chicken and chicken-mixed dishes, number four soda, energy drinks, and sports drinks, number five is pizza, number six alcoholic beverages, number seven pasta and pasta dishes, number eight Mexican mixed dishes, number nine beef and beef mixed dishes, and number 10, unheated organic nut oils.

This is shocking and reveals the problems we are facing with weight gain and obesity. The first four groups on the recommended list are loaded with sugar, fructose, and grain. If this is the diet you are following, we need to change that ASAP!

Sadly, this was actually the 2010 Dietary Guidelines for Americans and continues to this day. ***Unbelievable!***

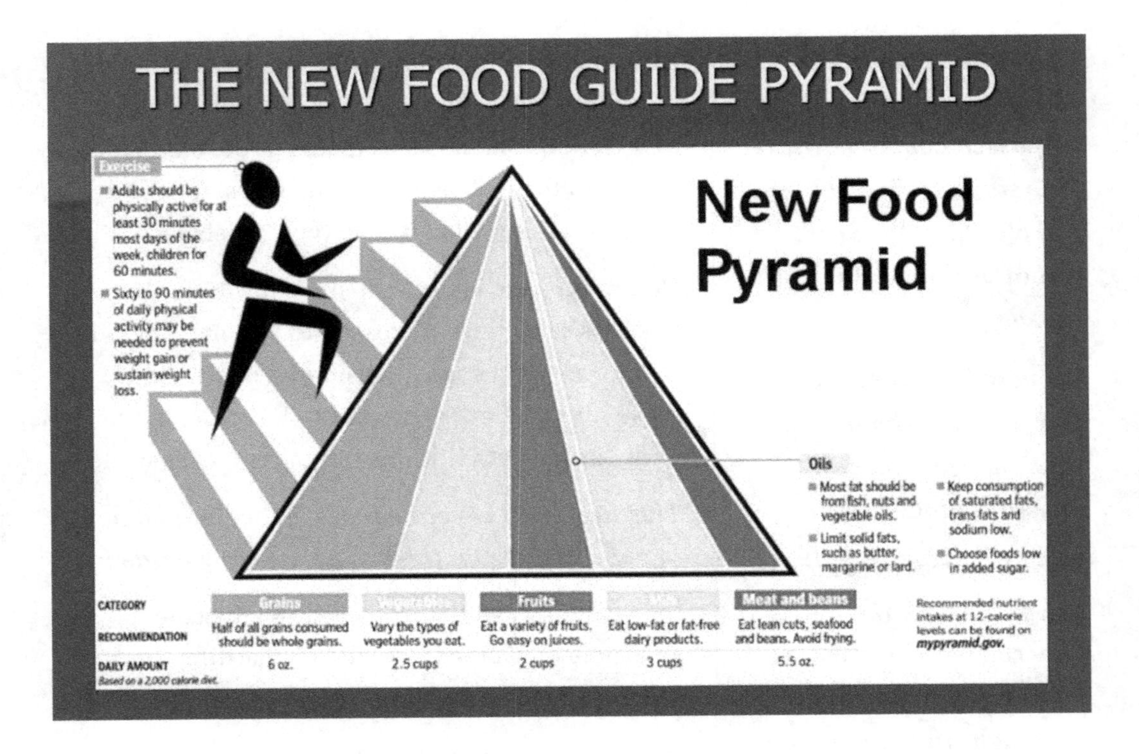

Have a look above at the government's New Food Pyramid and see under fats and oils, that they are telling you to limit butter and lard and instructing you to eat vegetable oils.

What you should be eating is olive or coconut oil, avocado oil, butter, and lard. Yes, I actually said lard! The second largest triangle represents dairy. Some dairy is good, but not fat-free dairy. Often fat-free foods are packed with sugar and fillers we cannot even pronounce, and stripped of all nutritional value. Even most shredded cheese in this country is mixed with sawdust! Supposedly this is to keep the cheese from clumping!

We are not going to eat fat-free anything unless the food is naturally fat-free! That tiny yellow sliver being shown on the New Food Pyramid is criminal! The oils from fish and nuts are okay, but then they go and instruct you to eat vegetable oil and limit butter or lard.

This is not good advice, and there is plenty of scientific research to prove it.

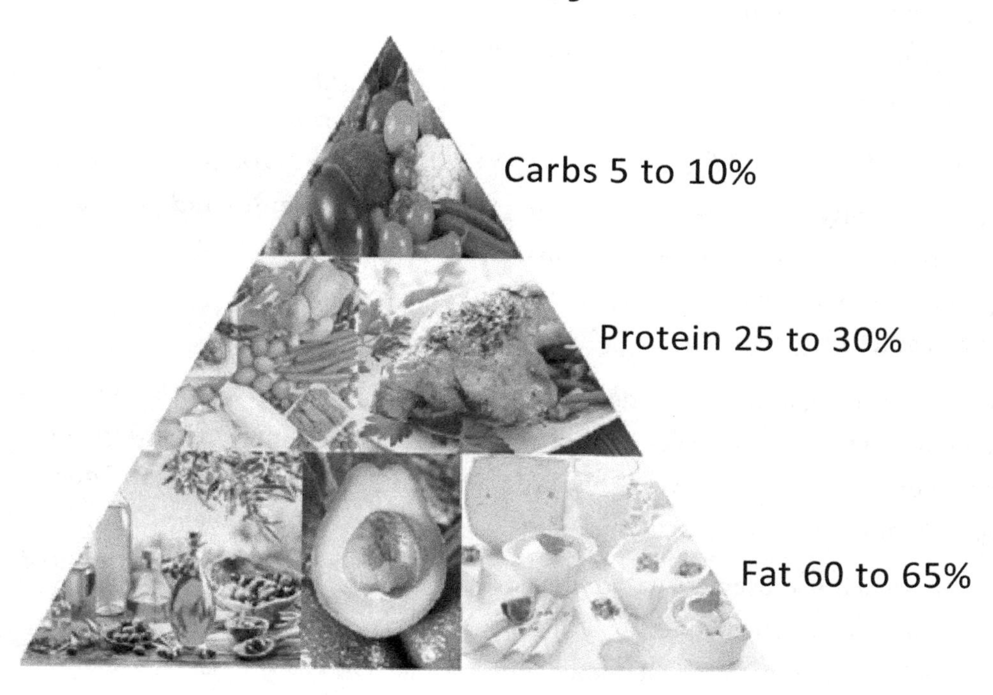

Barbara's Keto Pyramid

You will quickly see that my keto pyramid is considerably different from the government's New Food Pyramid as it shows absolutely no bread or whole grains. On mine you will get your carbohydrates from vegetables and some fruits.

Protein is next of importance, and is the middle section of my pyramid, providing adequate amounts to keep you satiated and energetic. It is also important for maintaining lean muscle, and a healthy brain.

My pyramid's foundation is built on fat, and the body needs plenty of it to provide energy and support a healthy brain. Fat is satiating to the body and enhances overall health of skin cells. Fat adds richness and flavor to food.

You may be asking, what does this have to do with me?

Well, everything if you are eating the current government recommendations for a high carb diet like my family used to do. If it had not been for the fact that we were so active working every day, we might have been overweight.

Let's fast forward forty years and have a look.

Most small family farms are a thing of the past, as they have been gobbled up by massive conglomerates where cattle no longer graze the pastures, and rarely even see the light of day.

Cows' udders hang to the floor engorged with milk from being injected with excess hormone, and have barely enough room to lie down. They are nothing more than milk-producing machines.

Chicken farms are a disgrace, with chickens existing in such crowded conditions they cannot get off their roost. Many die just a few inches from water because they cannot get through to the watering trough due to the crowded conditions. Many dead chickens are just left to decay on the floor until they look like dried up pancakes.

Other chickens walk over the bodies and even lay eggs in this putrid environment. They have been fattened up with genetically modified corn and soy and pumped up with antibiotics to such a degree that they cannot even walk, and their beaks have been cut off to keep them from pecking each other.

If you were living in this type of unnatural environment, you would peck at other chickens too!

An article written by Anahad O'Connor[7] for **The New York Times** ***on September 1, 2014, reviewed results of three separate diets tracked for a year, financed by the National Institutes of Health and published in*** Annals of Internal Medicine.

150 women and men were divided into three groups, one low carb group, one low fat group, and one high fat group. They were told the amounts of fat or carbs they could eat, but without calorie restriction.

The group losing the most weight were the 50 who were on the high fat, Doctor Atkin's modified diet. They could eat all the fat and protein they wanted with unsaturated fats, olive oil, fish, and nuts. They also ate cheese and red meat.

History and science do not support eating fake oils and fake foods made up of chemicals to be a healthy human.

I get absolutely furious when I think of all the suffering the government food pyramid has caused for innocent victims like my mother.

If the 1980, food pyramid is so healthy, why are so many people sick and fat? The 1980 food guideline has been a total disaster!

Chickens were meant to graze and peck for worms, grubs, and bugs, not be tortured in these deplorable conditions. Pig farms are another shocker. Pigs live in such squalor and are creating such noxious gasses do to this same corn and soy diet that no one can even live within a fifty-mile radius for the smell.

The conditions for these animals are deadly, so what do they do about it? Pump them full of antibiotics and hormones to keep them from getting sick and make them grow, that's what! How do these drugs affect you?

Take a look around at our current population and what do you see? Male breast, wheat bellies, hairy women, overweight children, and children aging faster and younger than ever before. Girls are entering puberty at startlingly young ages, and both young boys and girls have sprouted guts and breasts.

This is tragic, and the culprits are wheat, sugar, GMOs, and hormone infested meat and dairy. Infants are being fed soy formula which creates even more hormone. Is it any wonder we now have obese babies!

The antibiotics that are being pumped into our meat are criminal, as these drugs are then consumed by humans in meat, dairy, and eggs. No wonder we are all at risk of being antibiotic resistant, and superbugs threaten our very existence!

As the illustrious Dr. Phil, host of the Dr. Phil Show would say, "How's that working for yah?"

Looking at rising numbers of overweight and obese people, and the growing epidemic of heart disease and diabetes should answer the question. **It's not working!**

If this does not make you angry, it should! We need to fix this disaster and take charge of our amazing bodies and those of our children and grandchildren. The only ones profiting from this travesty are the doctors, hospitals, pharmacies, sugar producers and wheat growers, and the real drug lords of this country, the pharmaceuticals.

I watched a woman burst into tears at a drug store as her prescription cost had doubled. She couldn't pay the new amount of $375.00. This is another valid reason to fight back and stay well! You owe it to yourself and your body to read and research what is going on with your food.

Many countries have already banned Monsanto's weed killer, Round Up, as a potential cancer causing product, but unfortunately, thanks to the powerful lobbyists in Washington, Round Up is not banned in this country!

Nearly all corn, wheat, and soybean have been treated with Round Up. I was furious when I realized that the soymilk put out by Soy Silk, which I had been drinking for years, is genetically modified soy and heavily sprayed with Round Up. You even find this soy in baby food and formula! Now I drink organic almond or coconut milk.

The best way to tackle this enormous problem is to take charge of what you are buying and what is going into your mouth.

Once again I have to say, you must research and question everything you always took for gospel truth.

Take charge of your health and do not ever be intimated about questioning and speaking out when it comes to your health.

A high fat diet is still being demonized by the federal government—remember they are the ones who handed you this disastrous diet in the first place—don't be fooled!

The more we demand organic food, the more available it will become at cheaper prices. Tell your grocer every time you are there that you want organic food.

Read labels and buy organic whenever possible. I know it is more expensive to buy organic food, but by no longer purchasing the unhealthy sugar-laden high carb food you have been eating, you can now invest the extra cost in embracing your health!

Affecting their bottom line is the best tactic to getting the attention of the food producers and manufacturers. Whole Foods has been adamant in their commitment to carry as many natural organic products as possible. They also have a rule requiring any product genetically modified must carry a GMO label on the product.

Incidentally, I just read on Dr. Mercola's website, www.mercola.com that Monsanto has been ordered to put a warning on the Roundup packaging that their product may cause cancer. Even traditional grocery store chains are offering more and more certified organic foods.

Our local Publix grocery store now carries grass-fed hormone-free beef. Organic foods have not been treated with chemicals or been genetically modified. Organic beef cattle have been pasture raised and not fattened up with hormones and grain, and then, of course, their milk, crème, cheese, and yogurt are also hormone free.

CHAPTER TWO

SUGAR: THE #1 DEMON

CHAPTER TWO

Sugar: The #1 Demon

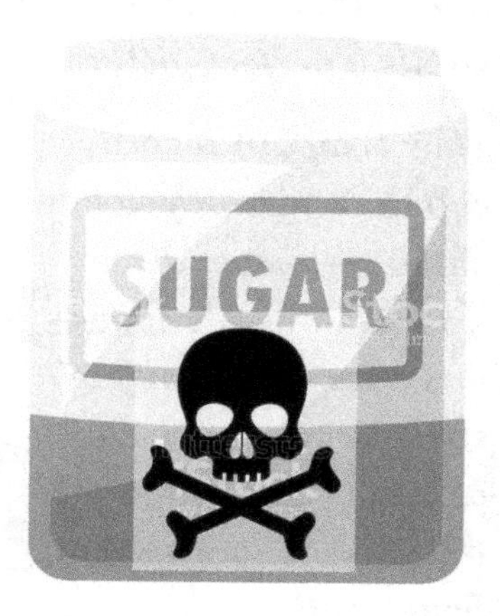

The number one evil in our food world is sugar. All bags of sugar should have a skull and bones poison label on the front of the bag with a warning that eating this product could kill you. Sugar has absolutely no dietary value whatsoever.

In 2012,[1] Jonny Bowden, Ph.D., C.N.S. and Stephen Sinatra, M.D., F.A.C.C., published a book titled, *The Great Cholesterol Myth, Why Lowering Your Cholesterol Won't Prevent Heart Disease and the Statin-Free Plan that Will.* I highly recommend this enlightening book. Interestingly, they target sugar as the main culprit in the American diet, even labeling it a demon.

Dr. Bowden and Dr. Sinatra discuss how hormones control what happens to food once you have swallowed it, determining if the food is stored as fat or gets shuttled for use elsewhere in the body. Enter insulin and its partner glucagon. Insulin's job is to build up, and glucagon's job is to tear down.

Their purpose is to support your blood sugar and keep it stable.

Insulin is a hormone and vital in controlling blood sugar as it regulates how the body uses and stores glucose and fat. It also keeps your heart free of disease, and your body free of diabetes.

Glucagon is vital to brain function and keeps blood sugar levels from going too low, which could cause death. It allows the body to regulate and utilize glucose and fats by stimulating the liver to break down glycogen to be released into the blood as glucose.

Insulin works in tandem with 5 hormones, including its main partner, glucagon, adrenaline, noradrenaline, cortisol, and human growth hormone. Insulin is the big gun in this hormone mix, and the other five just mentioned help to balance insulin's effects. Insulin's role is to keep the blood glucose levels in a normal range to help prevent diabetes.

High insulin levels narrow your artery walls requiring your heart to beat harder to pump the blood through. Insulin, your fat storing hormone secreted by the pancreas, is stimulated by sugar and as the cycle picks up speed, the fatter you get!

This creates a cascade of battles as insulin levels rise. You may now be well on your way to full-blown diabetes. According to the National Kidney Foundation, diabetes injures the small blood vessels in the body, which inhibits your kidneys from properly cleansing your blood. The body begins to hold on to more water and salt than it should, thus causing swelling and inflammation.

If your body could talk, it would now be screaming at you to stop the sugar load now! It may even become difficult to empty your bladder causing you to have to use a catheter. This is no way to live, and this book will teach you a better way.

Many who are diagnosed with diabetes will suffer from kidney failure. This results in perhaps a lifetime of kidney dialysis.

The risk for heart disease becomes greater as the body becomes inflamed and plaque begins to build up in your arteries. According to the late Dr. Atkins, inflammation can potentially raise your triglycerides and lower your good cholesterol.

According to Dr. Bowden and Dr. Sinatra, sugar is the number one enemy leading to heart disease.

One of their analogies paints a perfect picture.

They compare sugar to cotton candy—if you have eaten cotton candy or watched it being spun—it is pure sugar. Imagine sticky sugar molecules chugging through your blood, gumming up your body's cells.

The doctors then refer to the opposite situation—eating keto friendly protein. They use the example of oysters as pure slippery protein, sliding easily through your blood free of sticky glue-like sugar, doing their job.

Do you want pure protein easily zinging through your body, or gooey sugar clogging and choking your arteries like melted gummy bears?

I think we both know the answer to that question.

We are a nation of sugar lovers—from weddings, baby showers, birthdays, holidays, reunions, parties, entertaining—you name it, and we eat sugar.

Sugar used to be a special treat, but now it is an everyday event.

When I was young, I witnessed one of my aunt's crouching down between our stove and the sidewall in the kitchen. She was hiding because she was eating a candy bar.

As I stood there staring at her, she put her finger to her lips and said 'shhh.' She did not want to share the candy bar with her two kids. She then whispered, "I crave these."

I wanted to scream, "I want a bite too," as we never got our own candy bar, except occasionally at my Grandmother's house.

My mother just rolled her eyes and shooed me out of the kitchen.

I just had my yearly visit with my doctor to review recent blood work. I have a gene mutation called MTHFR, which interferes with my body's ability to process the B vitamins. This puts me at risk for inflammation and heart disease.

My doctor was totally shocked that my homocysteine level is low and no treatment was necessary. I was so happy I almost cried as most of my older family members have died from heart disease.

My triglycerides are now 54, and my HDL cholesterol is 133, which is a near perfect ratio, but it was not always that way. If your ratio is the opposite, according to the latest data, you have a big problem, and we have a lot of work to do to control inflammation in your body.

High insulin levels contribute to plaque in your arteries. The higher your blood sugar levels, the more insulin is secreted. Once your insulin levels are totally out of control, brace yourself for the dreaded diagnosis—diabetes or heart disease or both!

The body at this point is working in overdrive to get rid of all the excess sugar, and the only choice now is to deliver it to the fat cells. The big caveat here is the fat cells are possessive of their sugar and hold on to it making weight loss even more difficult. Insulin increases water and salt retention, setting the stage for high blood pressure.

According to Anne Alexander,[4] Editorial Director of *Prevention*, "The average American consumes 130 pounds of added sugar per year—that is, sugar that's an ingredient in food rather than sugar that is naturally occurring in food."

Recent research tells us that people deny the amount of sugar they consume, however, here is the kicker—most of it is consumed in their own home.

I was shocked to learn from Dr. Mercola that there is only one teaspoon of sugar per gallon of blood in your body, and if you added just a mere tablespoon more, you would die from hyperglycemic coma!

How on earth does your body keep this ratio in check?

Insulin is the hormone in charge of sugar control duty. Remember, wheat turns to sugar in your body, so mix that with all the sugar you consume, and you force your pancreas to pump out more insulin to protect you from sugar overload. The end result with the strain on your pancreas is insulin resistance with diabetes just waiting in the wings.

I cannot stress enough the delicate balance your body must maintain to protect you and keep you alive!

Let's take a closer look at the different types of sugar.

First of all, we have plain ole table sugar. This type of sugar is used for baking, sprinkled on cereal, added to coffee, etc., and is a combination of glucose and fructose. Then we have high fructose

Insulin controls your glucose.

Think of insulin as a microscopic taxi that delivers glucose to your cells via the blood. It is either used for energy or stored as fat.

As excess fat gets stored by insulin, the more obese you become. This is a vicious cycle as the liver has no choice but to convert excess glucose to stored fat.

Dr. Atkins in his book* New Diet Revolution, *states that the lower the levels of insulin, the greater chance of one surviving breast cancer. This is all the more reason to control sugar intake.

In their May-June 2016 issue, Harvard[6] published an article by Laura Levis, **Are All Calories Equal?**

The article reviews excerpts from Dr. David Ludwig's book, *Always Hungry.*

Dr. Ludwig says, "We know that excess insulin treatment for diabetes causes weight gain, and insulin deficiency causes weight loss. And of everything we eat, highly refined and rapidly digestible carbohydrates produce the more insulin."

He explains how excess carbohydrates spike insulin levels that can cause the enzyme lipase to be turned off. Calories get stored in fat cells instead of the blood. The brain then determines that you are hungry and need more food!

The vicious cycle continues to compromise your health and ability to lose weight.

corn syrup which is in nearly all processed foods, but mostly in sodas and juice. High fructose corn syrup is also made up of glucose and fructose, but it is highest in fructose.

Remember that glucose and fructose are both carbohydrates, and during digestion, sugar is released into the bloodstream. Higher levels of blood sugar cause the pancreas to release added insulin so glucose can penetrate the cells.

The end result if too much sugar is consumed, you start spreading out around the middle, especially if you are loading up on heavy carbs from soda, fruit juice, beer, sweetened yogurt, potatoes, corn, and bread.

According to Dr. Mercola of mercola.com, overindulging in sugar and grain can have an adverse effect on your brain as it becomes overwhelmed from high levels of insulin.

As insulin and leptin become disrupted, memory and ability to think can become impaired. Alzheimer's or dementia then becomes a huge threat. Brain and heart health are the foundations for the things that matter to have a healthy body and a fulfilling life.

It is not too late to start taking charge of your amazing body and how you treat it. Every morning before your feet hit the floor, thank your body for providing an amazing home for you to live out your life. Make a pledge that from this point forward you will honor your body with proper food choices and exercise. Your future depends on it!

Fortunately, our voices are making a ripple, and many food manufacturers are hearing our cry.

What is causing this small stir?

Their bottom line holds the key. If we don't buy their product, they panic and either try to deny or hide the problem, or they face facts and race to fix it. The handwriting is on the wall, and many companies are desperately trying to come up with a safe sugar replacement.

When the government first announced that we should all go basically fat-free, give up cheese, butter, and whole milk, it did not take the food manufacturers long to come up with another plan. Enter cardboard no-flavor fake food and destroy-your-heart-hydrogenated-oils. If they could figure out a way to take away our flavorful whole foods, they can also find a way to give it back!

I know I am not painting a pretty picture for those who are simply struggling with a few extra pounds, but it is far better to understand what your future could look like. Taking charge at this point is critical to your quality of life. This keto diet will help you take back the reins with a new knowledge of what is happening to your amazing body!

You are going to learn how to trade glucose or sugar for fat and gain more energy and satiety. Your body has been running on sugar for energy and we are about to replace that with heart healthy protein, fat, and healthy carbs. With one in five deaths attributed to obesity in the US, sugar may be the biggest player in the length and quality of your life!

Change your diet by controlling the food you eat and slow down the madness.

This gives the body a break from the onslaught of sugar roaring through the bloodstream and the pancreas, (the organ responsible for processing sugar), frantically looking for a place to dump it!

Just as the food and beverages you are consuming caused the crisis in the first place, let's look at food friendlier to the pancreas and the fat cells.

Choose fiber rich foods and slow the whole process down by swapping sugar and wheat for fat, protein, vegetables, and fruit.

CHAPTER THREE

SUGAR ADDICTION

"Lead your body toward health and it will willingly fall in step. Your body wants to be healthy and reach its full potential in order to preserve life—your life. When you are active and healthy, your body thrives."

— Barbara Miller

CHAPTER THREE

Sugar Addiction

I hear this statement frequently, "I just do not understand why I crave sweets so much. I open the pantry and grab a bag of cookies, chips, or candy without even thinking about what I am doing. I feel addicted!"

Well, sorry to be the bearer of bad news, but yes you are addicted. That was the intention of the company that formulated it. They knew exactly the right combination of ingredients to keep you coming back for more.

The reason you can eat that whole jumbo bag of salty, greasy potato chips is simply because there is zero nutrition, just like that box of cookies you just polished off.

Your body cannot tell your brain that you are satiated because with zero nutrition there is nothing to report, so you gorge and later lament with the old saying, "I can't believe I ate the whole thing."

Research by the Journal of the Academy of Nutrition and Diabetes, ***concluded that 73 percent of packaged foods in grocery stores contain added sugars. Sugar addiction is one of the main reasons diets fail. You can reduce your cravings for sugar, but it will take three to four weeks.***

Without nutrients, your body thinks you are starving. You have heard the old adage I am sure, 'A calorie is a calorie,' and I am telling you that is not true.

For instance, a calorie from a low fat cardboard cookie is not the same as a calorie from a chicken thigh. The body looks at the calorie from the cookie and says, "What the heck was that, I'm still hungry, give me more." It calculates the calories from the chicken thigh and says, "Okay, I'm happy, that was good, and I am satisfied.

When your body thinks you are starving, it slows everything down to conserve energy. Unfortunately, you become what we call a "couch potato," and sadly you begin to look like a "couch potato."

Harvard Magazine[6] published an article in its June 2016 issue titled, *Are all Calories Equal?* Dr. David Ludwig at Harvard Medical School specializes in endocrinology and obesity.

Dr. Ludwig[10] is against the belief that overeating causes weight gain. He believes it is the other way around and that getting fatter causes people to overeat, and thus gain more weight.

Dr. Ludwig points out that insulin plays a dominant role in weight gain, he says, "Insulin is the ultimate fat-cell fertilizer." He says, "When fat cells get triggered to take in and store too many calories, there are too few for the rest of the body—that's what the brain perceives. We think of obesity as a state of excess, but biologically it's a state of deprivation, or the state of starvation. The

The sad news with this scenario is that you got nothing in nutritional value to reward your body, but you sure did tally up a boat load of sugar, salt and trans fats, plus mega calories.

Oh, no need to worry about keeping score, your inflamed body will do that for you! It is vital that you understand zero nutritional value in the food you have been consuming.

You cannot feel satisfied when the body is lacking what it needs, so you keep right on eating! This is what the term 'empty calories' means.

No nutrition equals the body demanding more food.

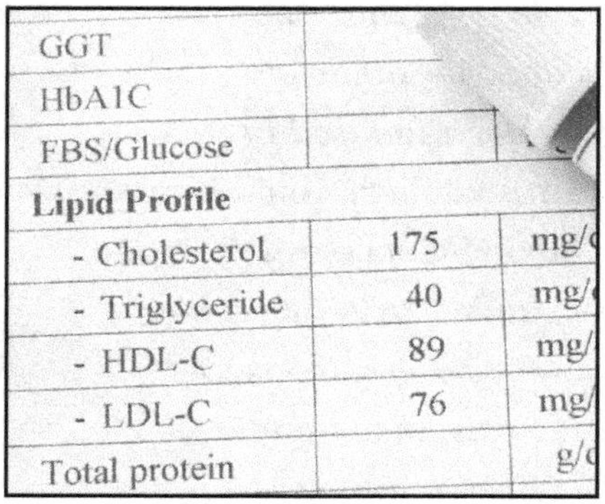

GGT		
HbA1C		
FBS/Glucose		
Lipid Profile		
- Cholesterol	175	mg/
- Triglyceride	40	mg/
- HDL-C	89	mg/
- LDL-C	76	mg/
Total protein		g/

Normal Lipid Profile

brain sees too few calories in the bloodstream to run metabolism, so it makes us hungry. It activates hunger and craving sensors in the brain, and slows down metabolism."

A major study conducted by Princeton University[8] comparing weight gain and high-fructose corn syrup revealed that rats fed high fructose corn syrup gained significantly more weight than those fed regular table sugar. The fructose corn syrup rats also showed increased triglyceride levels, which is a warning flag for heart disease.

According to psychology professor Bart Hoebel[7], who specializes in the neuroscience of appetite, weight and sugar addiction, "Some people have claimed that high-fructose corn syrup is no different than other sweeteners when it comes to weight gain and obesity, but our results make it clear that this just isn't true, at least under the conditions of our tests.

Professor Hoebel goes on to say, "When rats are drinking high fructose corn syrup at levels well below those in soda pop, they're becoming obese—every single one, across the board. Even when rats are fed a high-fat diet, you don't see this; they don't all gain extra weight."

The conclusion of this research project was that glucose occurring naturally in fruit was being processed for energy.

However, excess fructose was being metabolized to produce fat.

This is a warning to us that high fructose corn syrup is showing up in everything from soda pop to canned soup.

We just looked at a study comparing two groups of rats and the effects of fructose versus high fructose corn syrup.

Now we will see what happened in a documentary film produced by maker Damon Gameau[9] titled, "That Sugar Film." Mr. Gameau's goal was to study the health effects of a high sugar diet on a healthy body. Filming took place in Australia, and it is extremely revealing as to what happens to the body while consuming 40 teaspoons of sugar per day. This was actually the amount determined eaten by Australians at that time.

As of 2015, Americans consumed 23.5 teaspoons of sugar per day, and I am certain it is more now.

Much to Mr. Gameau's surprise, it was incredibly easy to consume 40 teaspoons per day, even though previously he consumed very little sugar. He quickly discovered that with one meal consisting of a bowl of cereal, fruit juice, and yogurt, he could reach his 40 teaspoons of sugar!

That is one meal, folks!

Gameau documented how rapidly his health declined as he began experiencing a "sugar high" followed by deep dive crash leaving him depressed, lethargic, and unable to concentrate.

It is vital that you consume sugar in moderation and in its natural form. According to SugarScience.org[11], sugar is added to 74 percent of processed foods and it is disguised under 60 different names.

Don't be deceived, and read labels carefully as if your life depends on it—because it does!

Following are a few of those names cleverly disguised in our food: Beet sugar, brown sugar, cane sugar, confectionery sugar, corn sugar, corn sweetener, corn syrup, dehydrated cane juice, dextrin, dextrose, fruit juice concentrate, galactose, granulated sugar, high-fructose corn syrup, honey, invert sugar, malt syrup, maltodextrin, maltose, mannitol, maple sugar, maple syrup, molasses, raw sugar, rice syrup, saccharide, sorghum, treacle, xylitol, and xylose.

Fruit contains fructose in its natural state; however, over consuming fruit can adversely affect insulin sensitivity. Remember, fructose is sugar, so control your fruit consumption. Make a list of what you eat each day, and you may be shocked at the sugar content, and then make a conscious pledge to start making healthier choices.

Many years ago, I used to frequent a little restaurant that also had the best bakery in town. I loved glazed donuts and would run in and order two glazed donuts and coffee to go.

I then retreated to my car where I could wallow in my decadent indulgence, especially if they were still warm.

Oh my! I can almost relive the experience by envisioning it in my mind. There was definitely something going on in my brain to make that experience so rewarding.

We now know that my brain was being stimulated to release Dopamine, creating euphoria of pleasure, even before I tasted my donuts! Dopamine is the neurotransmitter that drives you toward wanting the pleasure of food. As you consume more sugar, you become like the dope addict who needs to add more drugs to get the high they desire.

You are now a sugar high addict! What your brain really needs is healthy fat—not glucose.

Fast forward a couple of years after I had long given up indulging myself with a sugar treat. I was hurrying through the grocery store to grab a few items when I came to an abrupt halt. Straight in front of me was the bakery area, and you guessed it, the smell of freshly baked donuts waft through the air, and I could almost feel my brain light up and plead with me to please give it a fix of sugar.

It was letting me know that it remembers how good it felt to savor all that sugar! I stood still, closed my eyes and inhaled deeply, letting my mind experience a temporary sugar orgy. As I stood there groaning, I felt my face flush bright red as I sensed someone standing very close to me.

I glanced sideways, and sure enough, a man stood giving me that knowing grin. I hurried out as fast as I could, thinking how diminished he would feel if he knew it was only the donuts I wanted.

The food manufacturers are also on a roll, doing back flips to celebrate their new recruit into the ugly demon of sugar addiction. The more intense your feelings when consuming their sugar-laden food, the more times you will purchase it.

This lights up their life and fills their coffers. Jackpot!

The longer you continue down this path, the more difficult it becomes to make an about face and get off this downward path to obesity. Fat does not make you fat—sugar does!

In other words, the more weight you pack on, the control centers of the brain begin demanding more of that sweet stuff. As the feel good hormones are released, it becomes a greater challenge to win over the brain to a new program. The body and the brain are now at war.

According to Dr. Robert Lustig, The war on drugs has taken a back seat, but not because it has been won. Rather, because a different war has cluttered the headlines—the war on obesity. And a substance even more insidious, I would argue, has supplanted cocaine and heroin. The object of our current affliction is sugar. Who could have imagined

Your brain is having an orgy now with all the feel good hormones racing through your veins.

These are the same feel good hormones released during sex; the big difference is that nobody ever gets fat for having too much sex.

This is like being on drugs that your own body releases, which are actually opioids.

These release a host of emotions bringing intense pleasure and making you feel good—really good!

Stresses melt away, but guess what guys, the brain remembers and says, oh yeah, give me more!

You and your brain are now on a roll.

However, the irony in all this is that the roll keeps snowballing, and it ends up right on your gut, hips, and thighs.

More sugar?

Many have shared with me that as soon as they feel stressed, they grab a bag of cookies.

There goes that greedy active brain again lighting up like a neon sign that says—oh yeah—baby—cookies! You now become just like the TV character, "Cookie Monster."

My staff used to call me the "Cookie Monster," because I always had a stash of cookies in my bottom desk drawer, and when they were having a stressful day, they would raid my cookie drawer.

Real estate was a stressful business, and I sure bought a lot of cookies in those days. Along with my glazed donuts, cookies were the hardest thing I ever gave up.

Bye bye Chips Ahoy, Oreos, and my other best friend, Fig Newton.

something so innocent, so delicious, so irresistible... could propel America toward medical collapse?

We are learning more each day about sugar addiction and causes of obesity. A recent study from the National Academy of Sciences USA[12], using fMRI imaging scans on 24 volunteers to test their brain reaction to fructose versus glucose.

The results of the study were noted: *Parallel to the neuroimaging findings, fructose versus glucose led to greater hunger and desire for food and a greater willingness to give up long-term monetary rewards to obtain immediate high-calorie foods. These findings suggest ingestion of fructose relative to glucose results in greater activation of brain regions involved in attention and reward processing, and may promote feeding behavior.*

The importance of this study shows how fructose messes with the brains signaling that determines satiety. Fructose appears to encourage overeating and is in nearly all drinks and processed foods.

If your body does not get a heads up that you are full, you just keep right on eating. Fructose turns into body fat faster than other sugars, putting massive stress on your liver.

We have a lot of work to do in order to get the body and brain both working in tandem for total health and wellness to prevail. Please know that it can be done, and now that you understand how the brain and body communicate, you will be prepared to tell your brain that you are now running the show, and just like a child, it is not going to get any more sugar. We are going to get these cravings under control, and believe me when I tell you that fad diets of deprivation will not work! They have never worked before, and they will not work now!

There is no easy road out of sugar addiction, but you can do this, and the lifestyle eating habit in this book is your map back to finding health.

How did this happen to us and why hasn't someone stepped up to expose this terrible lie?

You say, "What lie?"

The lie the sugar industry perpetrated by paying reputable Harvard scientists to write a biased paper claiming that sugar was harmless and the real culprit was fat. This false report was made public 50 years ago and published in the *New England Journal of Medicine* in 1967.

Fortunately for those of us still living, the truth has finally surfaced through a researcher at the University of California, San Francisco. The research papers exposed that three research scientists were paid thousands of dollars to downplay any link between sugar consumption and heart health, placing the blame squarely on fat!

One of the paid scientists was D. Mark Hegsted, who was later employed by the United States Department of Agriculture to be its head of nutrition. He assisted in drafting the dietary

If you are under a lot of stress in your life and you have been rewarding yourself with sugary treats, you risk putting your desire for more sugar on auto-pilot, and then you become a real "Cookie Monster."

Remember, the food industry knows perfectly well that sweets are addictive, and they formulate exactly what they know will bring you back for more!

We are going to reconnect your body with the natural satiating foods it was designed to eat in order to keep you strong, healthy, and thriving well into old age!

A postdoctoral fellow at U.C.S.F., Cristin E. Kerns[13], discovered the documents in archives at Harvard.

The papers, written in 1964, purposed a plan by a top sugar executive, Mr. Hickson, to influence public opinion on the safety of sugar, "through our research and information and legislative programs."

The sugar industry provided the papers to the scientists and made it clear that they expected results favoring sugar.

Sadly, Harvard's Dr. Hegsted stated, "We are well aware of your particular interest, and we will cover this as well as we can."

It is a shame that the perpetrators involved in this treacherous act are dead and not here to stand accountable for their wicked deed!

guidelines for the federal government. Another Harvard scientist involved in the scam was chairman of Harvard's nutrition department. His name was Fredrick J. Stare. There was no disclosure to their connection to the sugar industry and that they were rewarded by the sugar industry for perpetuating one of the most deadly lies to the American people, causing illness, disease, and death. This very act was instrumental to ushering in low fat foods and deadly oils void of any nutritional value!

I believe this misleading advice is what killed my mother as she insisted that our government would tell us if sugar was dangerous! Well, Mom, they still haven't told us, but, some well-informed doctors have done their own research, beginning with the late Dr. Atkins, Dr. David Perlmutter, Dr. Robert L. Lustig, Dr. Mercola and Dr. William Davis.

Pedram Shojai[14], creator of well.org, authored an amazing book titled, *The Urban Monk.* In his book, Pedram also states that sugar is a drug and 10 times more addictive than cocaine.

He also states that sugar lights up our controls in the brain to make us crave more. *We're totally hooked on the stuff, and the fallout of this is starting to become apparent. It tweaks our blood sugar, lowers our immunity, triggers us to store bad fat, and feeds the bad bacteria in our guts.* Pedram explains that as long as we are overloading our body with nutrient lacking foods, we will always feel hungry and unsatisfied.

I remember watching a video of a famous diet guru yelling from the stage to hundreds of fans in the audience, "Fat makes you fat!" These are the exact words my mother used.

We have waited 50 years to have this lie exposed and saturated fat exonerated. Polyunsaturated and hydrogenated deadly oils have now been deemed as instrumental in causing heart disease.

In his *New York Times* best seller, *Fat Chance, Beating the Odds Against Sugar, Processed Food, Obesity, and Disease,* Robert H. Lustig, M.D., M.S.I., states, *if you had any residual doubt about "a Calorie is not a calorie," this analysis should remove any of it. Every additional 150 total calories per person per day barely raised diabetes prevalence, but if those 150 calories were instead from a can of soda, increase in diabetes prevalence rose sevenfold. Sugar is more dangerous than its calories. Sugar is a toxin. Plain and simple.*

It is not the calories but the source of those calories that matters.

If you have a fear of cholesterol, you may be happily surprised that according to an article published by the National Institute of Health, high cholesterol levels in elderly people showed better memory function.

I remember my own experience vividly as a former doctor insisted that I must begin a cholesterol lowering drug or face a heart attack. She could not accept the fact that my HDL or "good cholesterol" was 133. Evidently, because my HDL level is so high, it was questioned by the lab doing the

There was another doctor paying special attention to the high rise in cardiovascular disease and the connection to sugar. His name was Dr. Yankin, and sadly he passed away before he could convince other cardiologists that high sugar consumption was dangerous and possibly deadly!

In fact, Dr. Yankin called it, "pure, white, and deadly."

Similarly, Dr. Atkins tried in vain to impart that fat was not the enemy—a diet high in carbohydrates was the problem. Sugar and starches are high carbohydrate foods, in fact, white flour should have been listed with Dr. Yankin's sugar, as it is also, "pure, white, and deadly."

In Dr. Yankin's book,* Sweet and Dangerous, *he went so far as to insist that sugar should be banned!

According to Dr. David Perlmutter, MD, author of, *Grain Brain*, Nothing could be further from the truth than the myth that if we lower our cholesterol levels we might have a greater chance of living longer and healthier lives. Studies have also shown that there have been no fewer deaths from low cholesterol compared to high cholesterol. In fact, people with higher cholesterol numbers fared much better, living longer during the study.

testing, as above the 133 on the lab report was a notation, "verified by several tests."

Remember, this score is the result of my diet along with exercise. This lifestyle eating is the very eating plan I am presenting to you in this book!

Many large studies have attempted to prove that lowering cholesterol levels would lead to a longer healthier life by reducing heart disease risk. This is not true.

Let's take a look at what Dr. George Mann, a researcher with the Framingham Heart Study has to say. Dr. Mann says that the lower the cholesterol, the greater chance of heart attacks, and believes that individuals are being scammed and profit and pride are behind perpetuating this lie.

There have been multiple studies that debunk the theory that high cholesterol causes heart attacks. I encourage you to do your own research before you allow some uninformed doctor to prescribe cholesterol lowering drugs.

CHAPTER FOUR

WHEAT: THE #2 DEMON

CHAPTER FOUR

Wheat: The #2 Demon

Make no mistake about it, sugar and wheat are in bed together, and they are the health robbing bad boys on the block! They need to be driven out of town like the deceptive criminals they are.

We have already exposed some of the havoc sugar raises with your body, and we are about to expose its partner in crime, wheat. You will begin to see how both sugar and wheat influence high blood sugar levels.

Mike Geary[1], known as "The Nutrition Watchdog, is a Certified Nutrition Specialist, and bestselling author, and he has a lot to say about wheat and its impact on your body. Mike says wheat causes something called glycation in your body. These compounds called AGE's or Advanced Glycation End Products, actually speed up aging in your body. This can include damage to your joints, organs, and skin, causing wrinkling. Here it is again guys; *high blood sugar levels* can multiply and speed up age-accelerating AGEs in your body.

This is not a way to age gracefully. Remember, your brain, heart, liver, and kidneys are organs!

Mike says another major component of wheat is a carbohydrate called Amylopectin-A, and has been shown to spike blood sugar higher than regular table sugar. There they are again, the two bed-partners, sugar and wheat doing their best to mess up your body. Wheat causes your blood sugar to spike and remember what we said about sugar clogging up your arteries, well now it is teamed up with wheat!

This presents a potential disaster for you and your body as sugar and wheat race through your body like a runaway train!

Just as I have already mentioned, there is nothing good about sugar, and there is absolutely nothing good about wheat. If you really take inventory of the amount of wheat you consume, I think you might be shocked at the results.

Wheat, my friend, is in everything! Well, nearly everything, along with its partner sugar. Wheat and sugar are in most processed foods. Any food that is taken out of its natural form and put in a box or most cans has wheat and/or sugar added.

All deserts, cookies, crackers, Matzo bread, cakes, donuts, candy bars, thin mints, dinner rolls, whole wheat bread, white bread, croutons, English muffins, corn muffins, bagels, deep fried onion rings, pancake mix, pretzels, potato chips, corn chips, hamburger helper, soups, packaged mixes, ketchup, mustard, mayo, salad dressing, soy sauce, syrup, honey, and nearly all prepackaged marinades, soda pop, energy drinks, desert coffees, fake creamer, ice-cream, swirl fake ice-cream out of a machine, shakes, sodas, fudge bars, Dixie cups, Bomb pops, and the list could go on and on.

The giant food producing companies do not want you to become aware of their unethical practices, especially as it concerns whole wheat and its effects on the body.

Amylopectin-A is a carbohydrate found only in wheat. This is not a harmless carbohydrate, and it can drive your blood sugar through the roof, higher than pure sugar, and higher than any other carbohydrate.

There they are again, wheat and sugar doing their nasty number on your body!

Along with wheat speeding up aging through AGE's, wheat can also cause inflammation to joints and organs. As your blood sugar rises, the faster the AGE's are formed, the faster you age, and the spiking of insulin—equals added weight gain, joint pain and again wrinkled skin.

I know—right now you are wondering what in the world will I eat? No worries, we will get to that issue, and I promise there will be plenty to eat that will not only get your blood sugar and cravings under control, but your weight as well.

The more wheat you consume, the more insulin levels are affected, and your body now struggles to control blood sugar. This reaction to out of control insulin levels takes its toll on your pancreas, possibly leading to insulin resistance, and type-2 diabetes is lurking just around the corner. Weight gain begins creeping up inch by inch.

William Davis, MD[4], author of the #1 *New York Times* best seller, *Wheat Belly*, and *Wheat Belly Cookbook*, tells us what makes wheat different.

First of all, gliadin protein, the opiate-like compound that stimulates appetite is unique to wheat. No other food additive—high fructose corn syrup, GMO corn, sucrose, fat, food colorings, preservatives, etc.—stimulates calorie consumption like wheat. Eat wheat and increase calorie consumption by 440 calories per day, remove wheat, and reduce calorie consumption by 440 calories per day.

Yes, I said we were not going to count calories; however, these are empty, worthless calories that do massive damage to your body, and make you gain weight! Doctor Davis even goes on to say that two slices of bread increase blood sugar and insulin more than candy bars, and thus stimulates visceral fat or that nasty abdominal dangerous inflammatory fat.

Dr. David Perlmutter[2], author of *Brain Maker* says, *Visceral fat is more than merely an enemy standing by. It is an enemy that is armed and dangerous. The number of health conditions now linked to visceral fat is tremendous, from the obvious ones such as obesity and metabolic syndrome to not-so-obvious—cancer, autoimmune disorders, and brain disease.*

He relates a large waist measurement or hip to waist ratio, the smaller the brain's memory center, the hippocampus.

An article posted in *The New York Times*[3] by Jane E. Brody, on November 16, 2017, paints a dark picture of the dangers of weight gain. The article states: *Reviewing more than 1,000 studies, the International Agency for Research on Cancer and the Centers for Disease Control and Prevention linked the risk of developing 13 kinds of cancer to overweight and obesity, especially cancers that are now being diagnosed in increasing numbers among younger people.*

The study went on to say that the heavier you are, the greater your risk of being diagnosed with cancer.

My own experience with wheat, as I shared earlier, caused almost instant weight gain. As I already mentioned, many years ago, I read about a new diet that promoted eating a lot of carbs, mostly pastas every day. So I began eating more bread, linguini, spaghetti, penne, lasagna, stuffed shells, and pizza.

However, sadly, I did not lose a single pound. Instead, I gained 15 pounds, and where did these pounds go, you guessed it, right on my belly! Not only did I gain weight, but it seemed like suddenly I could not remember anything. I had terrible "brain fog."

Dr. Perlmutter explains that waist circumference is a predictor of health, and the greater the measurement, the greater the health of the brain is at risk.

The final result is a faded memory and an unsightly bloated wheat belly that can usher in a host of chronic health conditions.

Wellness is not a 'medical fix' but a way of living - a lifestyle sensitive and responsive to all the dimensions of body, mind, and spirit, an approach to life we each design to achieve our highest potential for well-being now and forever.

— Greg Anderson

As I began losing my curvy shape, I started to feel out of control. I developed a rash all around my hairline, and it was raw and irritated most of the time.

No matter what product I tried, nothing seemed to help.

I also started having irritable bowel syndrome with serious bouts of diarrhea followed by constipation. I suffered the most embarrassing problem of odorous intestinal gas. My abdomen was bloated and swollen most of the time, my clothes were too tight, and I was miserable!

I had started to develop a gut!

It was a problem for me to travel or even go shopping with friends because just like a current television commercial depicts a woman always scoping out the closest restroom, is exactly the way my life was at that time.

I wound up spending all of my time in the restroom and inconveniencing friends and family. My daughter said it was no longer fun to go shopping with me as she was tired of waiting outside the restroom door.

Finally, my poor sick body made it very clear that I needed to address this issue. I was in a local mall, and without warning, I doubled over in excruciating pain which seemed to radiate from my bowel.

I was close to my doctor's office, so I just walked in and begged to see him. It didn't take long for him to conclude that my bowel was having serious spasms that were causing my pain. He sent me straight to the hospital for x-rays, and the diagnosis was irritable bowel disease or (IBS).

They quizzed me and asked what I might be doing differently to cause this. I related how I had changed my diet to mainly pasta dishes. The attending doctor gave me a blank stare and said he did not know if that had anything to do with it, but would give me a prescription to calm things down.

Every time I researched IBS, I learned more about what causes this problem.

I learned that wheat allergy could cause raw skin irritation, which was what I had on my scalp and around my hairline. Once I eliminated wheat, the skin irritation went away.

I determined that dairy, such as; milk, cream, and ice-cream could trigger a reaction that sentenced me to hours in the bathroom. I had to be extremely careful about the lunch choices I made while dining out.

I also suffered from gastroesophageal reflux disease known as GERD. As soon as I would lay down at night, the discomfort started with acid burn that could only be relieved by curling up into a ball and forcing the gas buildup in my stomach to come up.

It was a nightmare as sometimes my food also came up and burned my throat. I still had not linked my IBS or GERD to wheat and sugar.

However, as more information came to light on the negative effects of carbohydrates and sugar on health, I began to get a clear picture of what was

Irritable Bowel Syndrome, or IBS, affects 10 to 15 percent of people in the U.S.

It is a miserable condition for some and grossly uncomfortable for others. The condition can lead to constipation or diarrhea.

One of my dear friends suffered from this syndrome for many years. She was afraid to go to lunch with friends or family, as she spent most of her time in the restroom.

As I shared, I also experienced this condition for years and had no idea that I had a lactose and gluten intolerance problem.

I suffered with IBS for at least 15 years.

I began reading articles about these symptoms and found only one article that said carbohydrates could cause these problems.

I decided to go back to my old diet and stop eating pasta dishes and see what happens. Oddly, just as the article stated, all of my symptoms subsided.

The pain stopped almost immediately, and the weight simply fell off. Our bodies cannot handle highbred modern wheat, and sadly, most of the population has absolutely no clue! Folks, this is tragic. We must all step up and be heard!

There is nothing about wheat that is good for you. In other words, wheat has no nutritional value whatsoever, unless you are a cow, or have four stomachs.

happening to me. I learned that much of the food I was eating was, in fact, destroying my health and that carbohydrate foods increase stomach acid.

Wheat is far more harmful than you may think, and Amylopectin-A, a carbohydrate in wheat, contains lectin, which causes gut irritation and phytates, which can prevent absorption of important minerals like iron and calcium.

If you are loading your body up with a steady diet of wheat, you run the risk of celiac disease, ulcerated colitis, Crohn's disease, diabetes, fatty liver, and irritable bowel.

This also puts a tremendous strain on your heart and encourages weight gain.

We began eating wheat ten thousand years ago. We were never intended to eat grass, and we are now paying the price—big time!

Dr. Davis calls wheat *the perfect poison.*

Okay, the 'healthy whole grains' we are being encouraged to eat do contain B Vitamins. However, our bodies were not designed to absorb vitamins through grain. In fact, grain leaves the body nutrient deficient.

Where there is a heavy grain diet, there is a serious nutritional deficiency. The wheat of our ancestors is not the wheat of today. *The American Journal of Nutrition* compares a slice of whole wheat bread to eating six teaspoons of sugar! The promoted 'healthy whole wheat' is among the highest on the Glycemic Index of almost all foods.

As insulin and blood sugar rise, your blood has to dump it somewhere. Welcome belly fat and fatty liver disease along with diabetes.

According to Dr. William Davis[4], author of *Wheat Belly,* 90 percent of obese patients have moderate to severe degrees of small LDL particles, thus the term "bad cholesterol."

However, Dr. Davis says, it is the LDL small particles, not the total cholesterol numbers that can cause your arteries to fill with dangerous plaque. Cholesterol is actually found in all your cells and attaches to proteins known as lipoproteins.

LDL is the culprit that can lead to a heart attack by lodging in your arteries. That is a good reason to refer to it as the "bad cholesterol."

Of course, the drug industry is having a heyday producing cholesterol lowering drugs to treat this epidemic for the sheer numbers of people growing in size daily. Large fluffy LDL particles do not pose the problem, it is the small LDL particles that cause heart attack or stroke.

HDL, on the other hand, is a hunter-gatherer as it scavenges your blood for excess cholesterol and transports it to the liver, which breaks it down and boots it out of your body. The key is to keep HDL levels as high as possible with 60 mg/dL being the base measurement. The higher you can raise your HDL the better.

Not only is wheat loaded with carbs, but 75% are in the form of Amylopectin-A, which converts to glucose rapidly and encourages the formation of LDL particles, they are small, dense, and deadly!

If you have been monitoring your cholesterol—you know LDL, or low density lipoprotein, is the bad stuff in risk factors for heart disease. However, LDL particles get a bad rap because their size can determine whether they will take residence in your artery walls or not.

You want your good cholesterol or HDL to be high, as the higher your HDL, the more protection you have against heart attack and stroke. HDL inhibits harm from LDL. The smaller the LDL particles, the greater your chances of having a stroke or heart attack!

The overall cholesterol score isn't what counts; it is your type of LDL and the HDL score.

Dr. William Davis states, "Diabetes is associated with a characteristic "lipid triad" of low HDL, high triglycerides, and small LDL, the very same pattern created by excessive carbohydrate consumption."

You definitely want your HDL score to be as high as possible.

Your cholesterol levels will be as good as the food you eat and the amount you move!

Many large studies have attempted to prove that lowering cholesterol levels would lead to a longer healthier life, but this is simply not the case. Let's take a look at what Dr. George Mann[5], a researcher with the Framingham Heart Study has to say, "The diet heart hypothesis that suggest that a high intake of fat or cholesterol causes heart disease has been repeatedly shown to be wrong, and yet, for complicated reasons of pride, profit, and prejudice, the hypothesis continues to be exploited by scientists, fund-raising enterprise, food companies, and even governmental agencies. The public is being deceived by the greatest health scam of the century."

There have been multiple studies that debunk the theory that high cholesterol causes heart attacks, and I encourage you to do your own research before you allow some uninformed doctor to prescribe cholesterol lowering drugs. Remember, I am not a doctor, and I am not advising you to stop any prescription medication. However, I am saying do your own due diligence and research, research, research!

Why the entire scuttle about gluten?

Many people believe if they do not have adverse effects from eating wheat, they do not have gluten intolerance. However, remember how we discussed today's wheat has no comparison to the wheat of 50 years ago.

Today's wheat is cross-bred and sprayed with Monsanto's Roundup. This process has dramatically affected the structure of gluten, making it foreign to the body, thus causing inflammation.

We talked about how the addictive nature of sugar can make you fat when you keep coming back for more? Well, according to an article in *Paleo Hacks News Letter,* wheat is even more addictive than sugar.

It also states in the report that in addition to the rapid sugar rush wheat provides, it also produces specific compounds that bind to morphine like receptors in the brain!

Many have turned to gluten free bread believing it's a healthy choice. Not even close! Don't believe it for a minute.

They are generally loaded with unhealthy flours that are even worse than traditional bread, such as, potato starch, corn starch, and tapioca starch. All of these deadly white powders have no nutritional value whatsoever!

You are not going to lose any weight by replacing regular bread with gluten free and your blood sugar will likely soar! You may even gain more weight.

Once type 2 diabetes has developed, your body has a serious challenge. One challenge is a greater risk of dementia.

Yes, diabetes ages your brain.

Your belly fat is affecting your health as it does not

According to Dr. William Davis, author of **Wheat Belly, Lose the Wheat, Lose the Weight, and Find Your Path Back to Health,** ***"Gluten is the culprit underlying inflammatory damage to the intestinal tract in celiac disease. People with celiac disease must meticulously avoid food containing gluten."***

Also, according to Dr. Davis, gluten flour is replaced with starches like; cornstarch, rice starch, potato starch, or tapioca starch. These supposedly gluten-free foods increase your blood sugar even more than wheat!

I urge you to read Dr. Davis's book, **Wheat Belly.**

He goes into great detail to explain the dangerous affects wheat and gluten consumption have on your body.

Say "No" to foods containing gluten.

Remember, we mentioned the dangers of AGE's; dementia is a real threat to quality of life and independent living.

Life is no longer just about you. Have you considered who will take care of you?

Not every family is equipped both financially and emotionally to care for a loved one with dementia, or as the brain begins to atrophy, full blown Alzheimer's disease.

Many unfortunately wind up in a nursing home as there is no one to care for them.

Cognitive decline and diabetes go hand and hand, and we don't welcome either one of them!

just sit there and look unsightly—it is active, but not in a way that is healthy.

According to an article by Joelle Reizer, March 10, 2015, posted by *Life Line Screening*[6], *Belly fat doesn't just sit idly at your waistline. Researchers describe it as an active "organ" in your body—one that churns out hormones and inflammatory substances.*

This active organ is believed to create fatty acids that affect the liver and promotes the production of LDL or "bad" cholesterol and triglycerides. This inhibits insulin in controlling blood sugar and ushers in insulin resistance.

Eliminating sugar and wheat from the diet will be the first step in reducing metabolically active belly fat.

There is a hormone called angiotensin that controls blood vessel construction, and can be affected by abdominal fat, which increases chances of high blood pressure, heart attack, and stroke. As triglycerides rise, your body becomes more inflamed and your chance of developing diabetes increases.

According to *Harvard Women's Health Watch*, the risk for Alzheimer's disease triples with a large belly, even if you have not gained a lot of weight, an expanding waistline puts you at risk. They recommend brisk walking and strength training. If you hate to exercise but love to dance, then by all means dance and do it often.

Studies show that dancing also improves memory,

helps control blood pressure, and reduces fat. So shake your booty!

According to the World Health Organization (WHO), people are getting fatter and sicker. By 2015, the numbers globally could reach as high as 2.3 billion.

We are past that now, folks.

This is not just about the health of individuals, but also the tremendous drain on the future of our economy. Robert H. Lustig, M.D., M.S.L., author of the *New York Times* best seller *Fat Chance, Beating the Odds against Sugar, Processed Food, Obesity, and Disease: The obesity is not the cause of chronic metabolic disease. It's a marker of chronic metabolic disease, otherwise known as metabolic syndrome. And it's metabolic syndrome that will kill you.*

My husband, David, is an avid pickleball player, and has cultivated many friendships on the court. One gentleman in particular, whom he had not seen in a while, appeared to have lost a substantial amount of weight.

When David commented on how great he looked and asked how he had lost so much weight, he said, "It is quite simple, I quit eating bread. My vitals were getting way out of whack, and my doctor wanted to put me on multiple of drugs. I did my own research and decided to buck up and eliminate bread and sweets, and I have lost 40 pounds in six months!"

This isn't magic, folks; this is what happens on a ketogenic diet!

Dr. William Davis, author of **Wheat Belly, Lose the Wheat, Lose the Weight, and Find Your Path back to Health,** ***says, "Ten pounds in fourteen days. I know: It sounds like another TV infomercial boasting the latest "lose weight fast" gimmick.***

But I've seen it time and time again: Eliminate wheat in all its myriad forms and pounds melt away, often as much as a pound a day.

No gimmicks, no subscription meals, no special formulas, no "meal replacement" drinks or "cleansing" regimens required."

According to Dr. Davis, when on a low carbohydrate diet, one automatically eliminates wheat, and the pounds roll off.

The exciting part is when you eliminate wheat and sugar, watch the pounds disappear!

Wellness is associated with happiness. When you're happy, you're feeling good in your mind and body. That ties into being healthy, eating well, and exercising regularly. It also ties into being excited about things - like getting up in the morning and having a healthy breakfast.

— Stella Maxwell

Dr. Ron Rosedale of the famous *Rosedale Diet*[7] states, T*he culprit in the ability to create adequate ketone levels is still, overwhelmingly, eating too many sugar-forming carbohydrates. People may think carbs like starches are perfectly fine to eat and that they will not prevent ketosis. But that analysis is wrong. It takes a mere 100 grams of glucose-producing foods per day—which can easily come from starches to prevent ketosis.*

Eating too many carbs will prevent ketosis and throw your body back into craving more carbs, especially sugar!

Avoid starchy carbohydrates to stay in, or reach, ketosis.

It is vital to produce sufficient ketones to maintain satiety, and the only way to do that is controlling carbs, eating high fat, and not binging on protein. If you eat only protein or too much protein, you will not reach ketosis.

Eating fat is the answer.

I know from my own experience as a postmenopausal woman, if I start consuming too many carbs, I start to feel bloated and constipated, and some of my pre-keto diet symptoms return. This is a reality check for me to get back on track quickly. When you are craving carbs, your body often just needs more fat.

When I first started a keto diet many years ago,

I did not totally understand the need to control the amount of protein I was consuming. I had no idea when consuming more protein than the body needs, converts to glucose.

That's right—sugar!

This will definitely keep you from the ability to reach ketosis. Yes, your body needs adequate protein, but not primarily protein.

Once you get clear on the value of the right amounts of carbs, protein, and fat, you will be on your way to ketosis and serious weight loss.

According to Dr. David Perlmutter, author of *Grain Brain: The body will naturally and wonderfully create ketones when carbohydrates are restricted, as long as there isn't an overabundance of dietary protein.*

Think of ketosis as the state your body is in when it is burning fat for fuel. The beauty of this state is that the body will use ketones as a fuel source instead of glucose.

CHAPTER FIVE

OUR BRAIN ON GRAIN

More and more studies are coming out relating to brain health in relationship to your gut.

New research says the gut and brain communicate with each other, and a healthy gut may very well equal a healthy brain.

Hippocrates, the father of medicine said, "All disease begins in the gut." How he knew that so many centuries ago is amazing.

We now know that our entire body is crawling with bacteria or microbes, which cover every square inch of our bodies, inside and out. Most, however, hang out in our intestinal tract.

The important part is that the good bacteria thrive in order to keep the bad guys under control.

Your health and vitality depend on a healthy balance to ensure a healthy microbiome.

CHAPTER FIVE

Our Brain on Grain

It is quite staggering the sheer numbers of bacteria who call your gut their home. In biology class, I was always amazed to learn about the role these various bacteria play in fighting off threatening viruses and preventing infections, scrutinizing the food you ingest for toxins, which helps out the liver.

When you destroy the good bacteria in your gut through your diet, you set the stage for a host of ailments, allowing the bad guys to take the reins. This can raise havoc with hormones and sleep cycles, which directly affect the health of your brain.

David Perlmutter, MD, author of *Grain Brain, The Surprising Truth about Wheat, Carbs, and Sugar—Your Brain's Silent Killers,* reveals the devastating truth about the effects of wheat, sugar, and carbs on the brain.

Dr. Perlmutter states that *The cornerstone of all degenerative conditions, including brain disorders, is inflammation, which can be triggered by carbs, especially those containing gluten or are high in sugar.*

He believes that the state of our health, including our brain, is not in the genes, but in the food we eat.

We certainly have been a clueless nation to the real

effects of grain on our body. I for one had no idea what it can do to our brain from mental problems to migraines.

I encourage you to read Dr. Perlmutter's book in order to fully understand the scope of the devastating effects of a brain on grain. He does not believe that brain degeneration is a 'rite of passage' into old age, but the effects of wheat or grain.

Dr. Perlmutter explains that when gluten hits the stomach, it is broken down into a mixture of polypeptides that can cross the blood-brain barrier. These polypeptides are able to bind to the brain's morphine receptor, creating pleasure and feelings of euphoria.

In fact, opiate drugs bind to the same receptor! He also states that wheat produces a greater surge in blood glucose than most foods. The question remains, are we putting our brain at risk for disease by consuming copious amounts of carbohydrates, especially through wheat?

Dr. Perlmutter says "Yes."

In consuming too many carbs, we run the risk of starving our brain by depriving it of fat for optimal health. Our brain thrives on fat! If anyone calls you a fat head, thank them!

Remember, grain is how they fatten up livestock. Fortunes are made on 'grain deals.' The entire world consumes grain and the powers that be want to keep it that way!

Take a stand and say "No" to grain and watch your health improve in ways you never dreamed

"Do the one thing you think you cannot do. Fail at it. Try again. Do better the second time. The only people who never tumble are those who never mount the high wire. This is your moment. Own it."

— Oprah Winfrey

You have probably heard the term 'metabolic syndrome,' but do you really know what it means to your overall health?

Remember we talked about abdominal fat as active and deadly!

Ladies if your waistline is over 34 inches, and gentlemen, if yours is 40 or above, you have abdominal obesity, a marker for metabolic syndrome.

The American Heart Association[1] (AHA) and the National Heart, Lung and Blood Institute (NHLBI) answer that question.

Marker #1

There are five health issues that can lead to metabolic syndrome and marker #1 is excessive belly fat giving you that notorious 'beer gut' or 'apple middle.'

possible. When enough people take a stand against grain and sugar, they will listen.

It is imperative that you understand the dangers you face when you adopt a daily diet of sugar and wheat. I also want to expose the real reasons behind obesity today and the steps you can take to get control of your life and body.

Now you know the main reasons you are packing on the pounds and the steps to take to shed that weight once and for all!

An article in the *New York Times* titled *Obesity and Diabetes Tied to Liver Cancer,* on October 14, 2016, by Nicholas Bakalar, states: *A large study found that body mass index, waist circumference and diabetes are all associated with an increased risk for liver cancer. Liver cancer is the sixth most common cancer, and its incidence has tripled since the mid-1970s in the United States.*

The study was done by the Cancer Research and involved 1.5 million participants. They discovered that obesity increased liver cancer risk 21 percent and 142 percent as B.M.I. increased. For each two-inch increase in waist circumstance, the risk of liver cancer increased by eight percent.

There are many slang expressions referring to the liver such as: lily liver; What am I? Chopped liver?; and the Elizabethans even referred to their monarch as the country's "liver."

Why all these referrals to the liver? An article in *The New York Times*[2], June 12, 1017, by Natalie Angier, titled, *The Liver: A Blob That Runs the Body* sheds some light on our amazing liver.

According to Angier, the Mesopotamians considered the liver to be our most valuable organ, even going so far as to declare that it is the seat of the soul and human emotions. Apparently, the liver is second in its duties only to the brain.

The liver is the gatekeeper and always on guard to evaluate what is going into your body. The liver has over 300 duties to perform, even controlling blood chemistry

The liver has the ability to repair and reproduce itself if injured. However, a new challenge to the liver is the barrage of foreign ingredients in processed food and drinks. There has been a surge in fatty liver disease and serious damage to this vital organ.

The caveat is that this super organ can only go so far in its efforts to save itself. If too much damage is done, a liver transplant is the only hope.

Marker #2

High serum triglycerides as a result of the sugar and wheat you eat in excess that winds up accumulating on your body. The majority ends up around your middle.

Your poor overworked liver desperately tries to store the excess triglycerides in fat cells, and you just keep spreading out. As your triglyceride levels rise, you are creating "The Perfect Storm" for a heart attack or

Corn is a grain, not a vegetable, used to fatten up farm animals.

Fatty liver disease is a serious condition. If the liver is compromised with fat totaling over 10%, it affects your body's ability to control blood sugar.

This can be exactly what has contributed to out- of-control triglycerides: fat from carbohydrates, not dietary fat.

The following is a quote from Dr. Eric Westman[3] from his book* Keto Clarity, *"The liver turns dietary carbohydrates into blood fat called triglycerides, and it's this fat that is stored in the liver. This is why corn, a high-carbohydrate grain that many think is a vegetable, is used to fatten up pigs and why it's also used to fatten the livers of ducks and geese for foie gras (which literally means 'fatty liver!'"

stroke—oh, and did I mention diabetes!

That fasting blood test your doctor has you do for your yearly exam will let her know if your triglycerides are at a dangerous level, or close to the top of the range of 150 milligrams. Your liver pumps out more triglycerides the more fructose you consume.

High triglycerides equal inflammation in your body. That inflammation can lead to heart disease and dementia. When your doctor writes a prescription to lower your triglyceride level, shake hands with metabolic syndrome.

Also, with your yearly blood work, your doctor will be looking at your cholesterol levels, the good, the bad, and the ugly.

Marker #3

If your good cholesterol (HDL) is sitting on the bottom of the deck, and the bad is on the top (LDL), you will undoubtedly be prescribed another medication to lower your cholesterol.

You may be asking, who dealt this mess anyway? Unfortunately, my friend—it was, unknowingly, you.

The lower your HDL, the more you begin to lose your protection to fight against plaque buildup in your arteries, and as the arteries narrow, your chances of experiencing a heart attack or stroke expands.

Marker #4

High blood pressure. If your blood pressure is high, your blood is being pushed with more force against the walls of your arteries and can damage your heart and potentially lead to plaque buildup and narrowing of your arteries.

You now may be diagnosed with coronary artery disease. You will no doubt be prescribed blood pressure medication.

Marker #5

If you are on medication because your fasting blood sugar is too high, you have just hit marker number five. Insulin resistance is the result of the body not being able to use its insulin properly, and blood sugar levels rise.

Once diagnosed with at least three of the five markers we have just outlined, you have metabolic syndrome and have placed your heart, brain, and body in serious jeopardy.

According to the National Heart, Lung, and Blood Institute[4], *Your risk for heart disease, diabetes, and stroke increases with the number of metabolic risk factors you have. The risk of having metabolic syndrome is closely linked to overweight and obesity and a lack of physical activity.* National Institutes of Health goes on to say that due to our rise in obesity, metabolic syndrome may surpass smoking as the leading risk factor for heart disease.

High blood pressure can be extremely dangerous and lead to a heart attack or stroke. No one feels high blood pressure—it is called a silent killer.

I resisted taking blood pressure medicine for five years and tried breathing exercises, aerobics and yoga.

I was shocked into reality when, at a routine exam, my blood pressure was 198/100. I was convinced it was 'white coat syndrome,' so I checked again as soon as I got home. To my shock, it was still 198/100. It was still high the next day.

Having a stroke would be right up there with the worse things that could happen. I now take blood pressure medication, and my blood pressure is in the normal range. Our local Publix supermarket offers free generic blood pressure medication with a prescription.

When functioning properly, Leptin prevents overeating and maintains a balance of energy.

According to Chris Kresser[5], New York Times bestselling author and alternative medicine teacher, high carb foods can lead to inflammation of the microbiota and can be a precursor to Leptin resistance.

Remember, we talked about empty calories and the body not being satiated?

Since Leptin's job is to let the body know you are full, and you do not need more fat. If you keep eating carbs, Leptin has no choice but to store more fat.

When it has no place else to store it, bingo—right on your belly!

It is important also to look at a hormone called ***Leptin*** and its role in fat gain. We talked about other key hormones and the role they play in hunger and weight gain, but Leptin is the "master hormone" of body fat regulation.

Dr. Stephen Guyenet[6], an obesity researcher, says somehow something changed in the brain's ability to communicate with Leptin to signal when you have enough fat stored and that it is safe to stop eating.

However, if the brain does not receive the signal, it thinks the body is starving. The brain sends out hunger signals to encourage you to keep eating and slows down the metabolism so you won't expend too much energy.

Leptin will, therefore, keep storing more and more fat!

Dr. Perlmutter states that, *Aside from sweetened beverages, grain-based foods are responsible for the bulk of carbohydrate calories in the American diet. Whether from pasta, cookies, cakes, bagels, or the seemingly healthy "whole-grain bread," the carbohydrate load induced by our food choices ultimately doesn't serve us well when trying to optimize brain health and function.*

Dr. Perlmutter also says that looking at the massive amounts of carbohydrates consumed, it becomes very clear why diabetes numbers are soaring.

Once the body becomes insulin resistant, the brain has difficulty blocking protein amyloids from forming brain plaque. Brain plaque is a major cause of dementia, or Alzheimer's disease.

KETO FOR LIFE

28 Day Fat-Fueled
Approach To Weight Loss

PART 2

TAKING CONTROL OF
YOUR LIFE AND HEALTH

CHAPTER SIX

EAT YOUR WAY HEALTHY

CHAPTER SIX

Eat Your Way Healthy

Now that we have exposed Demon Sugar and Demon Wheat, we need to banish them, and you are the exorcist! I will help you with this elimination process.

Start with the pantry and be brutal. This is the hardest part as it generally contains all of your baked goods, sugar, flour, crackers, cereals, cookies, candies, pancake mix, chips, popcorn, nasty oils, etc.

Grab that deadly heart destroying cooking oil and toss it. It will be replaced with heart healthy olive oil, coconut oil, avocado oil, flaxseed oil, butter, and lard. I know that stuff costs a lot of money, and it doesn't seem right to throw it all out, but it is destroying your health and future so get to it and pitch it!

You are not going to need these items ever again.

I am watching you, and I see you trying to hide that candy behind the coffee can—no cheating! We are going to replace these items with real nutritional food, most of which will be kept in your refrigerator, not your pantry.

Speaking of refrigerator, standing in front of the door won't fool me, so go ahead and open it. Let's have a look inside. Start with the margarine and pull it out, as we are replacing it with real butter.

I see the bottles of Coke and remember it is not the Jeanie in the bottle, don't let the disguise fool you. The Sugar Demon resides inside this bottle or any bottle or can of soda for that matter.

Pitch it!

Now for that orange juice that is supposed to be so healthy for you. Rubbish, orange juice is extremely sweet and loaded with sugar! If you are drinking skim or 2% milk, replace it with whole organic milk. When they take away the crème or milk fat, they take away the flavor, so sugar is added to pick up the slack.

Don't be fooled by the sugar demon trying to trip you up. Fat is not our enemy—sugar and wheat are the enemies.

The same is true for low fat or fat-free yogurt. Replace it with Greek whole fat plain yogurt. The whole cream or fat in the yogurt gives it a rich natural sweetness. Don't poison your family with artificially fruit-sweetened yogurt. It is loaded with added sugar, wheat, and soy.

I buy total fat Fage (pronounced Fa-yeh) which is an all-natural Greek strained yogurt. Toss in a few blueberries or raspberries for natural sweetness and flavor.

The first two weeks on this life-changing diet are the most critical. The very fact that you have now

I want you to eat well and enjoy the satiating flavorful foods you were meant to consume— not some sugar loaded nutrition lacking dish of poison.

You need protein and plenty of it, along with high quality fat!

You will get your carbs from healthy colorful vegetables and natural fruit.

Okay, I know you have been waiting for the skinny on this weight-loss plan.

You will love the yummy recipes and foods that will not only leave you totally satiated, but they are also easy to prepare and downright delicious.

We will look at ways to prepare your breakfast and lunch in advance so that you are not rushing out the door with only a cup of coffee in hand.

If you are busy preparing breakfast and lunches for kids and getting them off to school, you must prepare ahead of time or you set yourself up for failure.

It is imperative that we create a plan.

eliminated sugar, wheat, and grain from your diet, pantry, and refrigerator is a major change!

We have much work to do to get you to the point where you can stand in front of a full length mirror and say, "Damn, I look amazing!"

So, let's get started.

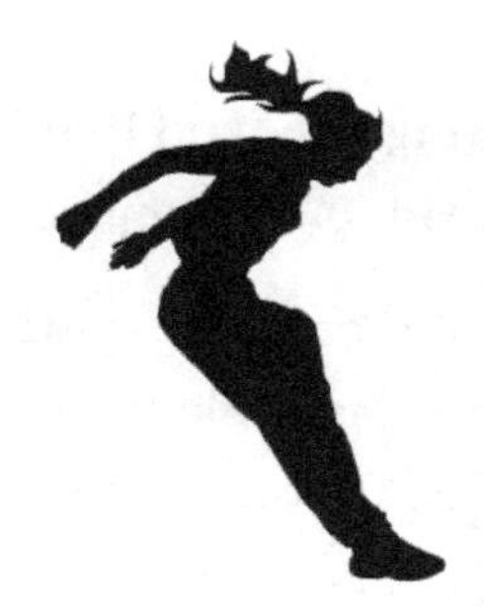

The Two Week Keto Jumpstart

During this two-week period, you will not be eating any fruit, with the exception of avocado, which we will eat plenty of due to its high fat content.

Not consuming fruit is actually putting your body in crisis as it will be screaming for sugar!

It is imperative that you replace everything you have gotten rid of by stocking your pantry and fridge with an arsenal so that you are never tempted to give up and order pizza! You won't be purchasing fresh or frozen fruit yet because you might be tempted to steal a little sugar fix.

No fruit for two weeks!

One of my coaching clients confessed that she had a tray of unbaked cookies in her freezer that she secretly kept, 'just in case.' She was having a major sugar craving and snuck to the basement where she kept her freezer and actually ate frozen cookie dough!

I am watching you, and that is a no-no! Get rid of all temptation.

Fill your refrigerator or freezer with fresh tomatoes, spinach, bagged lettuce, kale, collard greens, broccoli, cauliflower, peas, green beans, mushrooms, eggplant, red, green, and yellow peppers, squash and asparagus.

Frozen vegetables are a good buy, and they are generally cheaper than fresh, and freezing doesn't harm the nutrients. If buying fresh, refrigerate and don't overbuy as freshness degrade quickly.

Do not buy frozen vegetables with any kind of seasoning or sauce. They must be plain along with the frozen fruit.

It is critical that you eat enough dietary fiber or complex carbohydrates along with a high fat diet. Fiber fills you up while empty carbs leave you craving more.

Complex carbohydrates help the body feel satiated for a longer period of time as food moves through the digestive tract at a slower pace. Carbohydrates

Remember, your body is addicted to sugar like crack cocaine, and it wants its fix, and it wants it now.

Stand strong because sugar is no longer running the show—you are!

Some family members may be screaming for sugar and demanding to know what happened to the treats?

Just explain to them that what you are doing is life-saving and you need their support. If they are also struggling with weight gain, they may even join you in your challenge.

If your entire family is overweight, why not make this a family event with a contest that you all agree on.

Here's to your health!

By adding a variety of fruits and veggies to your diet, you will be replacing high carb processed food and those empty calories that have no nutritional value whatsoever.

The next important factor in the equation is to balance the healthy carbs with healthy protein and fat choices. I will provide menu choices and alternate suggestions so that you do not become bored and tempted to stray.

Hang in there champions; it is worth all the effort you can muster up.

I want to see you rock this!!

also provide valuable nutrients, vitamins, and minerals, which your body needs for optimum energy.

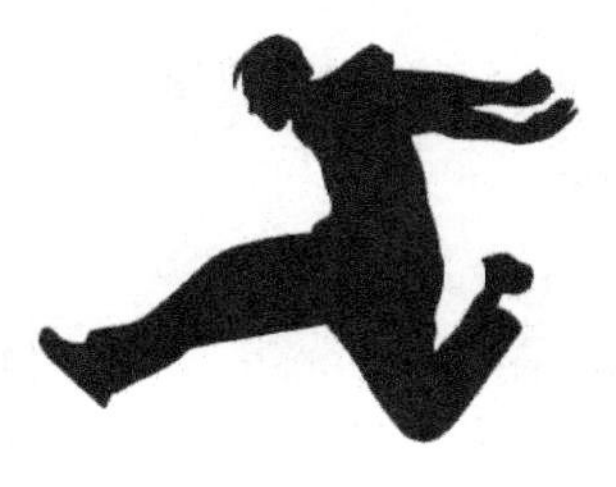

Here is a list of proteins that you may eat at any time.

PROTEIN

FISH: Bass, flounder, herring, halibut, mackerel, orange roughy, red snapper, salmon, sardines, sole, tilapia, trout, white fish, butterfish, anchovies, tuna fish and virtually all fish, and squid, which is actually a mollusk, *(if consuming calamari, it must be sautéed, grilled or baked, but not breaded. You may coat with almond or coconut flour). Avoid purchasing any seasoned or breaded fish. If you want a light dusting of flour, it must be coconut or almond flour. You may also coat with egg before coating with flour if desired.* ***Absolutely no wheat flour!***

SHELLFISH: Clams, crabmeat, lobster, mussels, oysters, scallops, shrimp.

FOWL: Chicken, Cornish hen, duck, goose, pheasant, quail, turkey.

MEAT: Bacon, beef, bison, bratwurst, ham, hotdogs, lamb, ostrich, pepperoni, pork, salami, sausage, veal, venison.

EGGS: Baked, deviled, fried, hard or soft boiled, omelets, poached, scrambled.

CHEESE: Blue cheese, cheddar, full fat cottage cheese, full-fat cream cheese, feta or goat cheese, Gouda cheese, mozzarella cheese, Swiss cheese. *(Do not overindulge in cheese as some have higher carbohydrate content).*

DAIRY: **(All of these products must be full fat with no added sugar.)* Butter, buttermilk, cottage cheese, ricotta cheese, sour cream, whole milk, yogurt, and whipping cream. *(Most non-fat or reduced fat dairy products have added sugar. When you remove the fat you remove the flavor).*

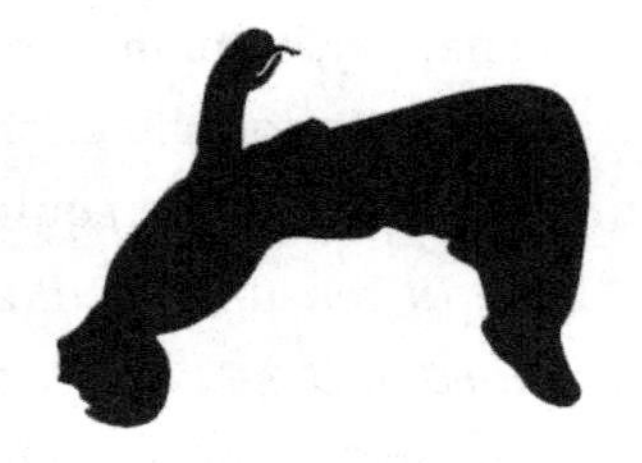

Here is a list of carbohydrates that you may have at any time.

CARBOHYDRATES

VEGETABLES: Arugula, asparagus, bok choy, broccoli, cauliflower, celery, chicory, chives,

You will also want some frozen meat choices like: steak, chicken, pork chops, pork sausage, veal, turkey, ostrich, bison, venison, ground beef, and seafood.

Whole Foods has the most amazing sausage patties made with organic sausage that are fairly spicy, but not over the top. You can also opt to buy organic ground pork and add your own spices.

Buy organic eggs when possible. You can even purchase boiled eggs in a sealed bag for a quick breakfast or snack, or even better, boil your own organic eggs. I like to keep baked chicken thighs and legs in the refrigerator as I often have a piece of chicken with my morning egg. It is not necessary to eat chicken breast unless you do not like the thighs and legs.

Remember, you want full-fat!

You can eat any protein for breakfast you choose.

Remember, first and foremost you need high fat and moderate protein.

The original Greek meaning of protein is "of first importance."

Bravo for the Greeks!

Back then the Greeks no doubt had plenty of fat from cheese and yogurt, and they were not trimming any fat off their meat. I am confident that they did not eat low fat anything!

Fat rules over protein and carbohydrates, and is necessary for fat loss.

Sorry Greeks!

cucumber, daikon, eggplant, endive, escarole, fennel, green beans, jicama, kale, leeks, lettuce, mushrooms *(all types)*, onions, okra, parsley, peppers, radicchio, radishes, romaine, shallot's, snow peas, sorrel, sprouts, summer squash, tomatoes. *(Avoid carrots, potatoes, parsnips, turnips, rutabagas due to higher carb content).* Once your weight is stable, you may have an occasional sweet potato.

FRUIT: Raspberries, strawberries, blueberries, and blackberries. (You may add other fruit after 28 days, but keep choices to a minimum until desired weight has been reached).

NUTS & SEEDS: Almonds, Brazil nuts, cashews, macadamia nuts, pecans, pistachios, sunflower seeds, walnuts.

FATS AND OILS

FATS & OILS: Almond butter, almond oil, almond milk, avocado, avocado oil, bacon fat, beef tallow, butter, raw coconut, coconut oil, coconut cream, coconut milk, chicken fat, duck fat, ghee, goose fat, hazelnut oil, lard, macadamia nut oil, mayonnaise, olive oil *(Avoid all vegetable oils including canola oil, and shortening as many have been highly processed and implicated in causing heart disease). Fat is your friend! Fake or highly processed oils are your enemy!*

Stock your pantry with canned tuna (oil or water), salmon, sardines, and chicken. (They even have these items in bags now, so if you are at a loss and running late, just grab a bag of tuna and your premade salad, and you are good to go.) However, a word of caution about the bagged seafood and chicken, I found it extremely salty, so check the salt level. I cannot stress enough the need to prepare ahead of time and be equipped to stay the course.

Buy frozen unsweetened fruit to have ready for your Four Week Daily Challenge, such as: blueberries, raspberries, blackberries, and strawberries.

Keep apples as a staple when you finish your two-week challenge. You can even keep a bag of apples and a jar of organic peanut or almond butter in your desk drawer to replace that bag of chips!

I still eat an apple every single day and often add a tablespoon of organic peanut butter or Almond Butter. My favorite is Santa Cruz Organic, creamy dark roasted peanut butter and Non-GMO verified. You can buy it on Amazon or at Wholefoods. The great thing about this peanut butter is the ingredients list, organic roasted peanuts, 1% or less salt, and no added sugar!

Okay, back to the apples.

They are a fiber-rich food and have many health benefits; however, they are on the high side of carbs. We will not be eating them in the first three weeks and only sparingly afterward until you stabilize your weight.

Buy organic if possible as most apples and other fruits are heavily sprayed with nasty pesticides.

It is imperative that you think of this diet as a dynamic trio!

This will consist of the three macronutrients which are fats, protein, and carbohydrates, and in that order.

We have all been trained to shun fat and eat high protein, but if you consume too much protein, your body will begin to consume muscle if there is no fat available.

Fat is used for fuel and energy on the keto diet.

A note about wine: Limit wine intake to one glass of red or white dry wine per day.

Avoid sweeter wines like Riesling. Sugar is actually added to many different wines, especially sparkling wines to enhance the taste.

Don't be tempted to cheat by adding a second glass as it adds more carbohydrates than you think, and will derail your progress.

Beer is totally out of the question as it is loaded with carbs!

If you absolutely hate wine, you may have one gin or vodka drink, however, do not mix with soda pop or juice of any kind.

Avoid mangos, pineapple, oranges, watermelon and bananas at this time as they are extremely sweet and thus have more carbs.

Once you have reached your desired weight, you can add these fruits occasionally to your diet.

Nuts are also a great snack such as: walnuts, almonds, cashews, macadamia, pecans, pistachios, and Brazil nuts.

Don't be alarmed about not getting fruit for two weeks as you will be getting natural sugar in some of your vegetables.

Our hunter-gatherer ancestors never had fruit or sugar on a daily basis. It was a special in-season treat, except when a beehive full of honey was discovered for a rare dessert.

Two Week Jumpstart Phase

You will be eating three square meals per day.

We will be taking your body through some major changes, and it is critical that you eat enough food to feel satiated or you set yourself up for failure. However, as your body is thrown into carb hungry crises, be prepared after a few days to sense massive carb cravings.

For my own experience, I felt tired, light-headed, foggy, and hungry. When I complained to my husband, who had lost several pounds on Atkins, he smiled and handed me six grapes! I just looked at him and screamed, "Six grapes, are you crazy, I am starving!"

He continued smiling and said, "Sorry honey, this is all you get, trust me when I tell you this will pass in a couple of days."

He is still alive, so I did not kill him, but at that point, I wanted to. I stuck with the diet, and sure enough, after two or three days, the cravings eased up and finally disappeared.

It is not easy to come off a sugar/carb high, but I did it, and so can you!

Week Three Phase Two Push

You should be in ketosis if you are eating enough fat and not overindulging in carbs and protein. Do not worry if you cannot tell if you are in ketosis or not; the most important thing is that you eliminate most carbohydrates. A ketogenic lifestyle is a process as you wean your body off wheat and sugar and adapt to a fat-fueled diet.

Week Four Power Phase!

Congratulations champions, you have made it to week four, and you are well on your way to taking charge of your weight! It is important to adapt to

Remember, vegetables and fruit are a healthy source of carbohydrates, and we need to balance carbs with protein and fat on this diet to keep you from craving sugar.

You will get enough in your salads and steamed or sautéed vegetables.

Don't skip your salad as this will be your main source of carbs in the first two weeks.

If you skip your salads, you will become constipated, tired, and miserable.

And that's not a nice place to be!

Dozens of Delicious Recipes start on Page 127.

I have provided dozens of recipes to keep you full and well satiated to encourage you to forge ahead and stay on course through Week Four Power Phase!

Choose your favorites.

No time to cook?

You can always substitute a steak and salad, or open a can of tuna and eat it with half an avocado and mayonnaise.

You must always remember to add enough fat, or you will fall back to your old diet and continue gaining weight.

the keto lifestyle eating to prevent gaining back the weight you have lost on "Keto for Life." Do not be discouraged if you have not lost the amount of weight you had anticipated as it is different for everyone. If you continue with low carb, high fat, and medium protein meals, your body will have no choice but to start shedding the pounds.

CHAPTER SEVEN

EXERCISE FOR HEALTH

CHAPTER SEVEN

Exercise for Health

Yes, you have to exercise!

I am an avid reader and researcher of health and wellness. Lately, I have been reading a lot of diet books, and to my surprise, readers are being instructed to stop exercising.

I will agree that exercise is not necessary to lose weight. If you are eating the right balance of fats, protein, and carbohydrates, you will lose weight without adding the exercise.

However, the problem with this is like some things in life that seem too good to be true; it eliminates many aspects of good health.

If you lose a lot of weight and never get off your chair, you will be sitting in a blob of loose skin and flab. It is vital to keep your body in motion to be healthy.

Exercise is mandatory for your health and well-being. In order for your amazing body to fight free radicals, plus keep you slim and calm, you must have a body in motion.

You have probably heard the term "oxidative stress," a condition brought on by stress to the body. In the book, *The Telomere Effect*[1], it classifies a free radical this way: *This noxious condition begins with a free radical, a molecule that is missing an electron. A free radical is rickety, unstable, and incomplete. It craves the missing electron, so it swipes one from another molecule—which is now unstable itself and needs to steal a replacement electron of its own.* This chaotic behavior races through your body robbing and plundering molecules to stabilize itself.

This act is an onslaught to your body. If not stopped by YOU, it can cause serious health issues, possibly leading to multiple diseases and we want to keep one of the number one diseases at bay.

I am talking about Alzheimer's disease.

In an article published in the February 2017 *Harvard Health Letter*[2], titled *What can you do to avoid Alzheimer's disease?* They stated that exercise could play a major role. *The most convincing evidence is that physical exercise helps prevent the development of Alzheimer's or slow the progression in people who have symptoms,* says Dr. Marshall. *The recommendation is 30 minutes of moderately vigorous aerobic exercise, three to four days per week.*

According to John Medina[4], affiliate professor of bioengineering at the University of Washington School of Medicine and author of *Brain Rules*, *It also slashes your lifetime risk of Alzheimer's in half and your risk of general dementia by 60 percent.*

You do not have to run a marathon, but you do have to move more than from a chair to the refrigerator and back. Keep your brain happy by

I recently read an article from AARP[3] from the Stanford Center on Longevity by Laura L. Christensen.

It stated that cognitive decline is not inevitable. The brain is in constant repair and renewal as long as we live.

The vital part of the equation is to keep moving!

I spent much of my life never having to worry about anything I ate. I was blessed with a tall, thin frame—until menopause came along.

Overnight I could no longer eat anything or any amount I desired, and I must admit I was shocked.

I had to take another view on comments from women who said, "I hardly eat anything and still gain weight." I used to think, "Yeah, right; I bet you are secretly chowing down."

What a rude awaking I had, and yes, I am ashamed at my insensitive attitude toward other women struggling with weight gain.

Here is the total truth: Unless you put exercise into the equation, you will never be totally in charge of your body.

providing adequate blood flow, and you will reap the benefits.

Exercise helps keep your brain from shrinking and keeps your brain synapse strong so you keep your memory. It is possible to even enlarge the brain with exercise!

The type of food you put into your amazing body is another step in developing healthy habits to keep you strong and fit.

The *Harvard Health Letter* says to eat a Mediterranean diet, stating that incorporating even partially to a healthy diet will help ward off Alzheimer's disease.

In case you might be thinking that because you are only 40 years old, you don't really need to worry about Alzheimer's disease. Well, think again because Alzheimer's actually begins years before it shows up in full bloom.

Now is the time to protect yourself and your future. According to Dr. Marshall, *The diet includes fresh vegetables and fruits; whole grains; olive oil; nuts; legumes; fish; moderate amounts of poultry, eggs, and dairy; moderate amounts red wine; and red meat only sparingly.*

I do not, however, agree with the whole grains. I have looked at the Harvard Food Pyramid, and it resembles the US new pyramid, which as mentioned earlier is heavy on grains.

Here is my easy plan to get you started on physical fitness to help improve your health, overall fitness and strength.

Want to get started on the road to physical fitness?

Then let's start with my 10/10 Change Plan: ten minutes of cardio and ten minutes of weight-bearing exercise.

Whether walking outside or on a treadmill, or peddling on an outdoor or indoor bike, the important thing is that you are moving. Start with an easy slow stride to give your body time to adjust and warm up, then gradually increase your speed to three miles per hour.

Do not attempt to begin by running, as you may injure yourself, and this is exactly what happens to some who try to run a marathon their first time on a treadmill. They literally cannot walk the next day and never attempt to exercise again.

My friend Karol shared this hilarious story with me that could have easily been a disaster. She was walking on a treadmill for the first time at her gym when for some reason as she was increasing the speed, she let go of the handles. She flew backward at the speed of light with her bottom leading the way. Fortunately, she landed on her bottom instead of face down on the treadmill. The only thing injured was her pride. Be very careful when first walking on a treadmill—and hang on!

Now is a good time to get moving!

If you start easy and do not try to tone up and slim down overnight, you will soon be on your way to better health and vitality.

If it fits in your budget and you can at all swing it, do hire a trainer. Even if you can only manage one or two sessions, it will be worth it. They will teach you the proper way to hold and maneuver weights so you will not have muscle strain or other injuries.

Always check with your doctor before starting any type of exercise. If you are suffering from body stiffness and pain, talk to your doctor about physical therapy.

Many people are not aware that their Medicare will pay for this so why not take advantage of it and get help moving!

In my early days of speed walking, I had read that if you pump your arms in a slightly bent position, parallel to the ground about waist high, it will tone the backs of your arms. Well, I am telling you, do not even think about it. I could not move for days, and my rib cage felt like someone used it as a punching bag!

My sister, Carol, told me her story of an overzealous try at walking. She started walking slowly and decided that if she put three-pound weights on each arm, it might help her get in shape faster.

Well, that went all right the first few days, so she thought maybe it would even be better if she strapped weights on each ankle. By the time she had walked one mile, she was so exhausted that her gait became a slow motion drag. She barely made it home before collapsing.

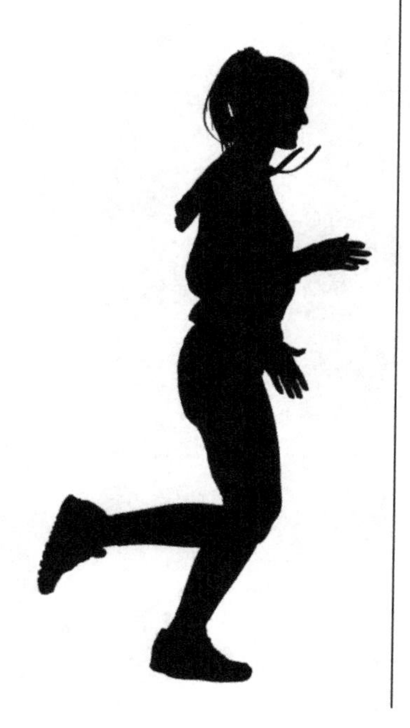

The next day, she could not move. She injured her neck and back and was unable to resume walking for a month. I tease her about why she did not hide the weights under a tree and come back with her car to retrieve them.

Start out walking easy; no weights strapped to your body!

The point in sharing these stories is to stress the importance of beginning slow and easy. You do not have to be a bodybuilder or marathon runner to get your body in shape. The important thing is that you get moving and reclaim your health and energy!

Once you have gotten into a routine and you feel comfortable, pick up your pace. Who knows, you may love the wonderful invigorating way you feel after a long brisk walk, and may decide to try running.

I enjoy walking and love being out early as I live in Florida and it can get very hot later in the day.

If you want to reshape and strengthen your body, incorporate weight lifting into your schedule. Start with two to three-pound weights and go easy on yourself.

I am currently participating in a Group Action class at one of the MVP gyms in my area, and it is definitely active. My husband speculates that we are the oldest ones in our class. We do everything from vigorous step aerobics to weight lifting.

I lift two 10 pound dumbbells, and my husband lifts two 20 pound dumbbells. I am not suggesting that you should do this, just that you should do something!

Do free weights only every other day so that you do not over tax muscles. If you only manage three times a week, that is fine, as long as you are consistent, you will see a difference.

"There is no passion to be found playing small - in settling for a life that is less than the one you are capable of living."

— Nelson Mandela

20/20 Change Plan

If you are physically able, now is the time to push your body a little bit more. You know it feels good, so move it! Twenty minutes of weight-bearing exercise and increasing your walk time to twenty

Remember, there is a wonderful fringe benefit as you increase your exercise time; you will also be releasing more happy hormones called endorphins, serotonin, dopamine, and oxytocin.

These hormones not only make you feel good emotionally, but they are morphine-like substances that help reduce pain in the body naturally, and the good news is you do not need a prescription!

I think we all need to go for a little jog!

This helps explain why body aches and pains actually can decrease when we increase our aerobic exercise.

minutes is a choice you will be happy you made.

Your body needs exercise to look and feel its best. Aerobic exercise that gets your heart pumping like dancing, biking, tennis, swimming, or walking will help give you a longer healthier life, to name just a few.

No one wants a life of stress, pain, and disease. Working your body, in turn, works your heart, helps reduce blood pressure, and oxygen intake is increased.

It's a win-win for your mental well-being and your body.

Getting the blood pumping, flooding your body with oxygen, can improve your good cholesterol (HDL), and reduce the concentration of LDL or low-density lipoprotein. Keeping your blood pressure to what your doctor feels is safe is paramount for your health and well-being, and aerobic exercise holds the key!

We do not want to be old and dependent on mental decline, pain, and taking a myriad amount of drugs just to stay alive. No, we want active minds, strong bones, mobility, and reduced risk for strokes, heart disease, diabetes, Alzheimer's disease and cancer. I have already done my exercise early this morning, but after writing this, I feel like I should go out and do it again.

Like I said earlier,
I not only want to be alive,
I want to live!

30/30 Change Plan

If time is a major issue, you may have to get up an hour earlier. Yes, I have no mercy and neither will your body if you do not treat it as a valuable entity that helps provide a quality life for its owner. Try to devote at least three days a week to the 30/30 Change Plan. You will be excited as you not only see your body change, but feel it as well. Adding muscle mass to your body will begin to replace fat, plus it will do wonders for your overall look and confidence. Muscle mass also speeds up your metabolism and helps with insulin sensitivity, giving you more energy and vitality. You can visit my website and click on the exercise tab at the top to see the exercises I have posted there for you. They can be done with light weights and are designed to help you start out nice and easy. The real bonus is you can pick up some weights from any sports store and do the exercises in the privacy of your own home! It is always best to check with your doctor before beginning an exercise program.

Many of the aches and pains that initially kept you from exercising in the past will diminish or disappear completely. Your energy level will return, and your posture will improve. Oh yes, and your skin begins to tighten around your frame, allowing your clothes to fit your new wonderful body. It is glorious to have your "skin fit!"

Time yourself to a fifteen-minute pace for your walk. This will give you two miles in thirty minutes. If you have added running or jogging

"Yoga is at the core of my health and wellness routine; even if it's only for 10 to 15 minutes I find it helps me to re-center and to focus as well as improve my overall core strength."

— Miranda Kerr

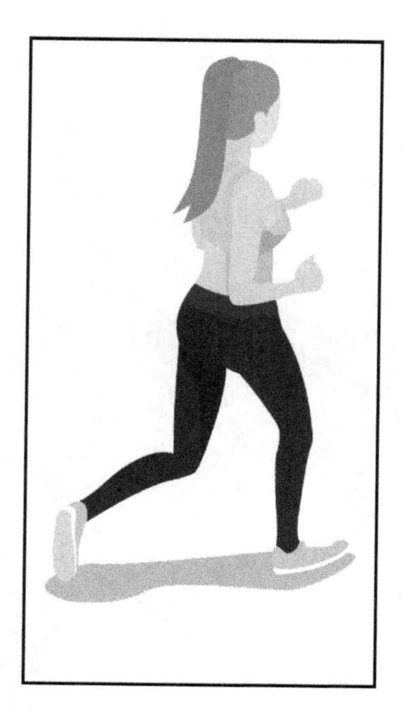

to your routine, you may even get in three miles. It is not necessary to run to get good results, so be careful not to risk injury. It is always best to check with your doctor before starting any exercise program.

Weight-bearing exercise will increase your lean body mass and help get rid of fat. Staying strong wards of cardiovascular disease, our number one killer, and helps us keep our independence. Women are most vulnerable to osteoporosis after menopause, but weight-bearing exercise helps maintain strong bones.

I invite you to go to my website at: http://www.BarbaraAndCompany.com and click the bar at the top that says Health and Wellness. You will see exercises I am doing that you can copy and use to help you get started with free weights.

CHAPTER EIGHT

HEALTHY LIFESTYLE

Don't be one of those people who join a gym during a hyped up moment after you just got bad news from your doctor who suggested you needed to start an exercise program.

Perhaps you decided this year you were going to get in shape and make a New Year's resolution to lose 30 pounds. You convince yourself that you will go to the gym tomorrow, but tomorrow rolls into next week, and now you lose interest and revert to old familiar turf—your couch in front of the TV.

What is that sitting in your lap? Sure does resemble a jumbo bag of chips and you look set to "eat the whole thing!"

CHAPTER EIGHT

"To get up each morning with resolve to be happy is to set our own conditions to the events of the day. To do this is to condition circumstances instead of being conditioned by them." — Ralph Waldo Emerson

You must be clear and precise in your mind as to what you want, and maintain unwavering focus with positive intent on achieving it! All your goals for your life are created on the inside, and then manifested on the outside. Once you grasp the truth of this statement, your whole thinking changes.

This is how you create your reality from the inside out, and where divine inspiration comes from. What do you want to manifest in your life? Having clearly defined goals can also provide clarity and purpose to your life.

Self-care is an absolute must. Eating a healthy diet and scheduling down time will go a long way in helping you stay on top of your game. Get adequate rest and spend time in nature. Walk, run, ride your bike, just find a meaningful way to keep moving.

There are wonderful fringe benefits when you exercise; you will be releasing those feel-good hormones called endorphins. They make you feel good emotionally, but they are also morphine-like substances that help reduce pain in the body naturally.

This helps explain why body aches and pains actually decrease when we increase our aerobic exercise. Your body needs exercise to look and feel its best. Start planning today for a healthy tomorrow and make the necessary changes to be the very best you possible. Make quality of life for you and those you love your number one priority. It is never too late to create change in your life! Allow success to flow through you.

I recently moved to a new area and joined a gym right away as I did not want to neglect my body for too long and break my habit. Even though I had been exercising my whole adult life, I still felt awkward going someplace entirely new.

I did not know a single soul so I immediately purchased a training session so I could learn the proper way to use the high-tech machines. It really enhanced my comfort level in a strange place where I knew no one.

I suggest you go to a group class such as yoga, Zumba, group ride, step aerobics, or if you have joined the YMCA, they generally have great pools for water aerobics.

You may have a friend or relative who is interested in joining you.

It is much easier to challenge each other than to go it alone! Let's not forget neighborhood walk, run, or cycle groups. Most local malls have walk groups and would welcome you to join them, especially if your climate is not always conducive to outside sports. As long as you are moving, it doesn't matter where you do it.

Yes, joining a gym is a motivating factor, especially when you have to sign a contract for a year and pay whether you go or not. However, it is not motivating enough because you must be mentally prepared to show up.

Write it in your schedule as a top priority. I highly recommend that you make an appointment with a trainer, possibly the person who signed you up, for a personal training session. You always have a first-time appointment to be shown around and introduced to the machines and various group classes available.

Take advantage of it, but then tell whoever you are working with that you want a personal training session for a half hour or full hour to help you work on targeted areas of concern. They will be more than happy to train with you or find someone who will.

The cerebral cortex, the brain's outer layer grows thinner over time.

Since this is the area where information is processed, and decisions are made, we need to protect our brain.

Well, the good news is studies have shown that those who meditate have a thicker cerebral cortex. Think of how you get bored just sitting around; well so does your brain get bored.

Hopefully, you are not keeping your brain in a "yawn state."

Get Brainy

Your body is not the only thing that needs exercise to stay fit. Your brain also needs a healthy workout.

Those who have careers and daily work challenges show less mental decline than those who sit home in front of the television most of the day and night. Staying mentally engaged plays a major role in warding off dementia. No, watching television is not active stimulation; it is passive and does nothing to preserve cognitive function.

Have a group of friends over and play bridge. This way you not only challenge your brain but you get the health benefits of laughter and interaction. Studies confirm that having a social network of friendships plays a major role in overall mental function.

Close friendships can even affect our immune system and reduce illness, such as the common cold, and help reduce blood pressure.

A study by researchers at Rush University Medical Center[1] in Chicago, Illinois, showed that you could counteract the effects of Alzheimer's disease by having goals and purpose. Having meaning and interest in your life can reduce cognitive decline by up to thirty percent.

Even if you already have early signs of Alzheimer's disease, having a positive attitude and living a purposeful life promotes cognitive health.

I have also been studying social media at home on my computer, so I can make better use of it to promote my books. There are so many new and exciting social media sites online that I have to limit just how many I want to spend time learning and visiting.

There is absolutely no reason to sit around bored with your brain in neutral. Take a computer class or buy a smartphone and actually learn how to use it.

You can even learn how to play numerous games on the internet. The brain loves anything new that challenges it to think.

Consider it like calisthenics to strengthen and give your brain a workout.

Butt Out

Quit smoking; it's a no-brainer.

It is not just your business if you smoke, it is the business of everyone you come in contact with. The impact your habit has on your children could influence them to mimic you and start smoking.

Even though I never smoked a day in my life, I now have scarred lungs which, my doctor believes, is the result of second-hand smoke.

Your second-hand smoke can harm everyone around you; not to mention what happens if you become ill.

I have had a lifelong love affair with learning new things, and am currently studying health and wellness through an online college.

This is a great way to wake up your brain and pull your thinking cap out of mothballs. Learning new information will help prevent cognitive decline.

The old* use it or lose it *still applies, and your brain loves to be stimulated.

Your brain will actually shrink if you do not use it.

Our bodies change as we age, and so does the brain.

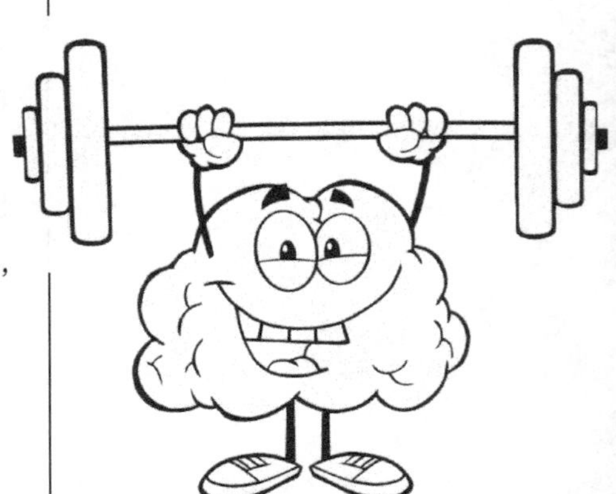

Smoking deeply affects your heart and lungs.

My father smoked three packs of Camels a day and died at 49 years of age from an aortic aneurism.

The first question the doctor asked was if he smoked.

Smoking narrows the blood vessels and compromises blood flow throughout the body.

Smoking can even cause bladder cancer many years after you have quit, and it is also a risk factor for periodontal disease.

My mother's sister, my Aunt Lillian, died of lung cancer. Aunt Lillian was beautiful, but her deadly habit of two to three packs of cigarettes per day cost her dearly. She was very independent, never got married or had children, and never saw any reason to quit smoking because it was "her business," and she enjoyed it.

Well, guess what, it was no longer "her business" when she became too sick to take care of herself, and my mother and family had to take turns caring for her.

Do yourself a favor and quit before it is too late to undo the damage.

Get Some Zzz's

Sleep deprivation is a growing concern in our modern world. There are so many distractions that keep us pumped up and hyped up that it seems nearly impossible to calm down and just plain relax.

Our homes are like an arcade—with flashing computers, televisions, cell phones, digital clocks, sounding beepers on our appliances. Help me, please! It is no wonder our circadian rhythms are all messed up. The body doesn't know if it is morning, noon or night; whether to wind down or get primed for a busy day.

I have struggled with insomnia for the last ten

years, and I truly sympathize with those of you who can't seem to get enough sleep.

I have started practicing Mindfulness meditation, and it has made a tremendous difference in my ability to go to sleep and stay asleep. I was only averaging four hours of sleep per night.

I could not seem to quiet my racing thoughts enough to relax and fall asleep. I spent the majority of my days exhausted and foggy. It was like running on half empty and in slow motion. Those of you who suffer insomnia are familiar with this feeling.

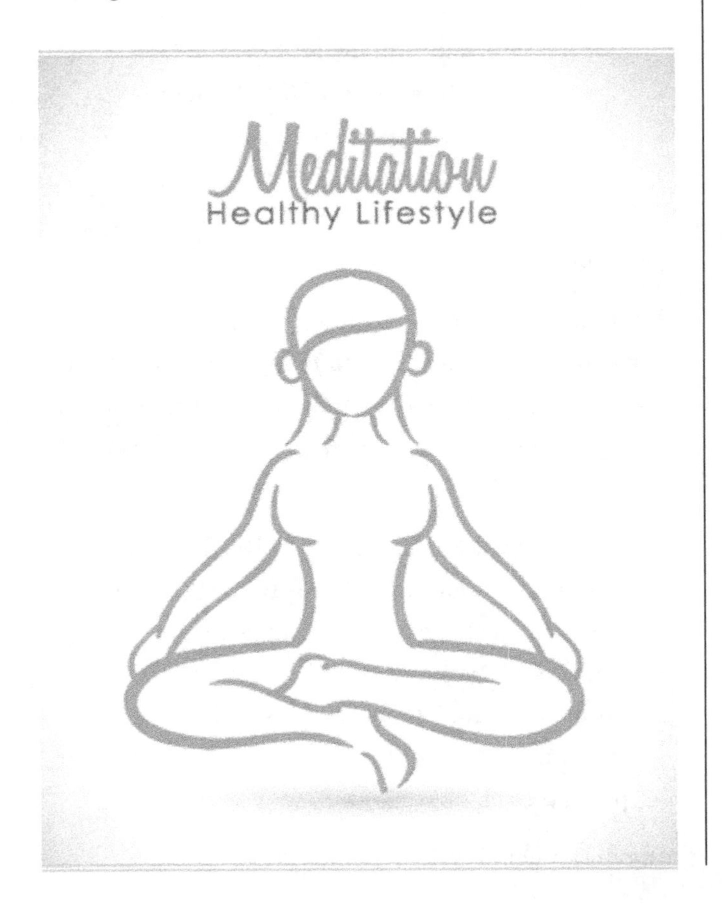

I highly recommend gentle yoga and meditation. The most important thing you can do is find what you might enjoy and just do it!

CHAPTER NINE

WEIGHT LOSS EQUALS WHAT YOU EAT

EAT CLEAN
DRINK WATER
STAY ACTIVE
BE HEALTHY

Foods high in protein help control appetite by keeping you satiated and feeling full.

Studies have also found that phospholipids in eggs can help calm inflammation in the body, as well as, lowering risk of cardiovascular disease by assisting the body in breaking down fat.

CHAPTER NINE

Weight Loss Equals What You Eat

Some of you are already surprised at being encouraged to eat the foods our government has been promoting against for 50 years. Even when their stand against healthy foods has been proven wrong, the discovery is announced in such a quiet, obscure way that it often goes unnoticed.

For instance, when numerous studies proved that cholesterol was no longer a concern for heart disease and we were free to eat eggs—again that great news was announced in one sentence.

Even when partially-hydrogenated and polyunsaturated oil was proven to cause heart disease, they are still touting the benefits of margarine to be healthy.

Many doctors are now stepping up to support these findings in an effort to help patients regain their health and wellness.

Many foods are repeated in the recipes that follow, and there is a reason for this—they are healthy and speed up weight loss.

Avocados are a big player in the keto diet, along with avocado oil, olive oil, garlic, cheese, eggs, cream, sour cream, broccoli, cauliflower, nuts and nut flowers, berries, and coconut cream.

Eggs

The incredible edible egg! It is so wonderful that one of my most favorite foods has finally had the cholesterol stigma lifted. Even though the government announced that cholesterol was no longer a concern for heart disease and we were now free to eat as many eggs as desired, I never stopped eating them in the first place.

My daughter Alison was raised on 'eggies' (as she called them). Apparently, eggs can raise good cholesterol (HDL), as well as, boost the size of LDL particles into a fluffier, good size.

Remember, it is those nasty small dense LDL particles that can lodge in your arteries and cause heart attacks. Eggs are loaded with healthy B vitamins that help support the nervous system.

Eggs also contain choline, an essential nutrient for cognitive function, in other words, eggs support your brain.

Amino acids are essential to life, and the body needs 20, but can create only 11. Fortunately, the amazing egg boasts of 9 amino acids which play a crucial role in protecting the health of the body such as; weakness, muscle wasting, and decreased immunity. Lutein and zeaxanthin are found only in the yolk of eggs, are two important antioxidants in their protection against macular degeneration and cataracts. Consuming these two antioxidants is vital in helping prevent blindness in the elderly.

Sunshine is not the only way to get vitamin D, yes, I am saying that eggs are a source of vitamin D, which supports bones and teeth, and even aids in boosting metabolism.

Who would have guessed that all this and more is packed into this oblong little goldmine known as the egg?

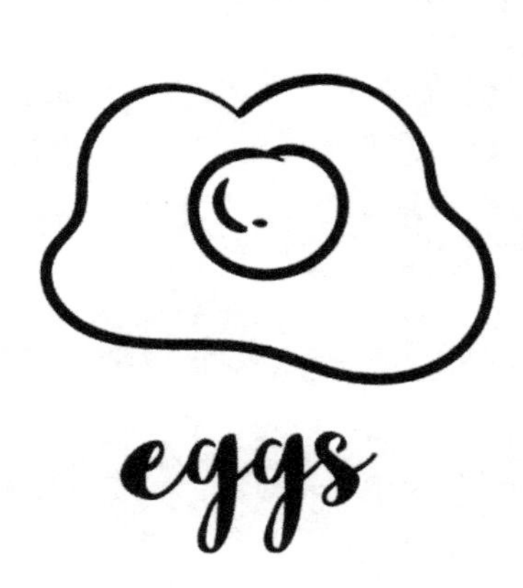

Avocados are the real "Jolly Green Giant."

Yes, they are loaded with fat; however, healthy fat can help you lose weight and help lower bad or (LDL) cholesterol. This fat is monounsaturated oleic acid, sound familiar; it is the same fat that is found in olive oil.

Carrots are not the only food that boasts of carotenoids, which help fight skin cancer; avocados are loaded with it, primarily in the outer darker green layer closest to the skin or peel.

Nearly all the essential vitamins for the body are contained in this super healthy green fruit.

Wow, so many impressive reasons to eat an avocado every single day. I do!

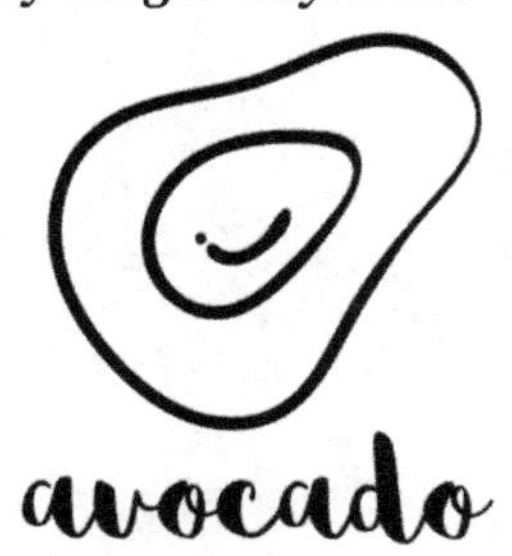

Avocados

Avocados are known as one of the most powerful foods for your health. They are loaded with photochemical compounds that can even aid indigestion through anti-inflammatory compounds.

This creamy, luscious fruit is a healthy source of omega-6, which is vital to the brain and central nervous system, and provides nearly 20 vitamins and minerals.

Surprisingly avocados are high in B vitamins, especially folate, which is vital for pregnant women to prevent birth defects. You won't find folate in most food, but it is abundant in avocados!

Vitamin C also takes up residence in avocados, even boasting 15 mg in a cup. Vitamin K deficiency plays a role in many diseases, especially heart disease, but it is also found in the skin of avocados. Vitamin E is a common addition to most one-a-day type vitamins, but vitamin E in avocados is superior and even aids in the health of your skin by helping prevent free-radical damage.

A study reported in January 2013 by The Journal of Nutrition and Cancer[1&2], revealed the power of photochemical found in avocados could aid in cancer cell death.

Remember, foods that are high in fat and low in carbohydrates actually aid in weight loss. Make avocado your daily vitamin regimen and eat your way to health.

OLIVE OIL

Olive oil has been around for thousands of years, and is actually a fruit chocked full of monounsaturated fat. Olive oil is a staple for those living in the Mediterranean basin where olive trees originated.

Olive oil plays a major role in the Mediterranean household, not only for cooking and salad oil, but as lamp oil, beauty products for skin and hair, bath soap, and medicinal purposes as an antibiotic.

Olive oil is one of the most heart healthy oils available and can actually lower bad (LDL) cholesterol while at the same time maintaining good cholesterol (HDL). Studies on the brains of mice showed better connections and less memory loss on those fed extra-virgin olive oil, compared to those not consuming olive oil. Brain inflammation also improved with olive oil.

A study by researchers at Columbia University Medical Center in New York[5], on 2000 people learned that those who ate closest to the Mediterranean diet lowered their odds of getting Alzheimer's disease. Olive oil was a major part of their diet and maybe reduced brain inflammation.

All the more reason to embrace olive oil and its many health benefits!

I suggest purchasing olive oil from California as the growers have stringent guidelines and strive to get the California Olive Oil Council, Certified Extra Virgin (COOC) seal on their labels, along with NON GMO Project VERIFIED seal.

While visiting Spain many years ago, I attended a lecture about olive oil.

The gentleman said that during past wars, many Spanish people had no food except bread and olive oil and how important it was to their survival.

He went on to discuss the many uses and benefits of this amazing oil and why olive oil is considered healthy.

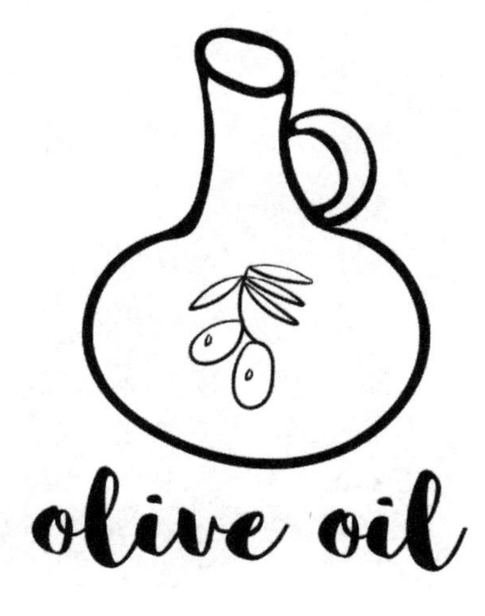

I highly recommend California Olive Ranch First Cold Press Extra Virgin Olive Oil, and it is available at most grocery stores for ten to twelve dollars. It is amazing with all the healthy certifications plus the olive oil is made and bottled right at their ranch here in the USA!

When I first went to Napa Valley Wine Country many years ago, my husband David and I had lunch in a beautiful olive grove at one of the wineries. The scent was amazing, and when we inquired as to the purpose of the small olive grove, they said the entire land had been a large olive grove and when wine became so popular, they burned down the olive trees and planted grape vines.

It is so exciting to see that they are once again embracing olive trees along with grape vines and fortunately they are producing the highest quality olive oil. See what happens when the demand is there, the producers step up to the plate and give us the quality we deserve.

CHEESE

Cheese is a powerhouse loaded with the vital nutrient B-12 which aids the body in neurological function. Cheese is very high in protein as well as fat which leaves the body feeling full and satiated.

According to an article published in the Journal of the American Heart Association, cheese can have a positive effect on the body by lowering bad LDL cholesterol. Cheese also contains calcium which aids in building strong bones.

Most are aware that cheese is loaded with bacteria, however, it is fermented which causes a healthy effect on the gut. Cheese not only affects the gut, but also the mouth due to a bacterium found in cheese called *Lactobacillus rhamnosus* that may protect against cavities.

A study done in Sweden and also posted in the *American Journal of Clinical Nutrition*[3] followed over 900 French men for several years. The good news is that those who consumed two ounces of cheese daily lived the longest during the study. Cheese contains calcium which aids in building strong bones. Researchers believe high calcium in cheese may help lower blood pressure.

Cheeses that are high in fat like sharp cheddar and Brie contain a fatty acid called conjugated linoleic acid, which is an anti-carcinogen, and may protect against heart disease.

It looks like there are plenty of good reasons to make cheese a daily staple in your diet.

According to studies in the* American Journal of Clinical Nutrition*, the risk of type 2 diabetes may be lower in daily consumption of cheese.

Fermented dairy also contains Vitamin K2, which may help the body from absorbing fat by moving it out of your gut.

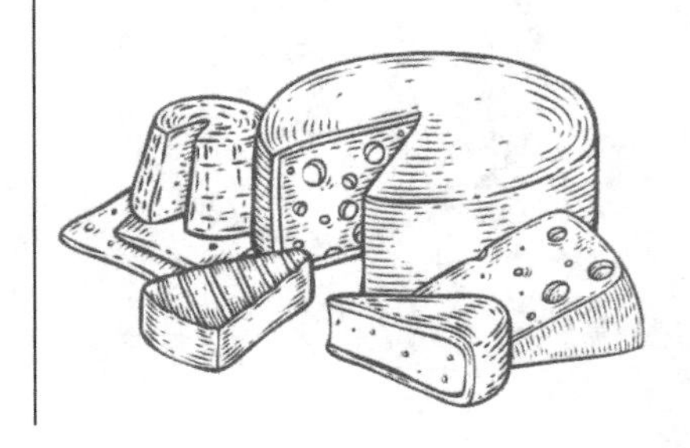

GARLIC

Garlic was known in ancient times to enhance health and vitality.

Garlic is related to scallions, onions, and leeks. Garlic is known as the 'Stinking Rose.' Those of us who eat garlic daily know if we breathe directly in someone's face, they will quickly take a step back. The sulfur compounds are a result of the active ingredient, photochemical allicin, which may be responsible for the health benefits of garlic due to its antiviral and antibacterial protection.

However, apart from garlic's pungent flavor and aroma, it has multiple compounds that may play a role in its healthy reputation. Dr. William J. Blot[4] of National Cancer Institute reported on large studies of people in China and Italy that showed a low rate of stomach cancer in those who consumed a lot of garlic and its relatives, onions, scallions, and leeks.

Garlic seemed to enhance the benefit when consuming fresh vegetables and fruit.

However, there are warnings for those on blood thinning drugs, which when consuming too much, garlic might interfere with the efficacy of these medications, and cause bleeding as it reduces blood clotting. If you are being prescribed anti-coagulant drugs, it is best to consult with your doctor on the risk of consuming garlic.

ONIONS

Onions are part of the allium family along with shallots, scallions, leeks, and chives.

Onions are known to have anti-bacterial and anti-inflammatory effect in the body. Some people can handle raw onions without stomach distress, while others can only eat them cooked.

Onions add such a healthy benefit to the body, and I encourage everyone to give onions a try, even adding it to soups and salads.

Onions aid the body in producing vitamin B-12, vitamin C, B6, iron, folate, and potassium. Onions are rich in the antioxidant flavonoid quercetin, which aids in preventing disease.

Onions, like garlic, may help prevent stomach cancer and produce more HDL or the good cholesterol.

There are multiple reasons to include onions in your daily diet.

I love hamburger salad, with a larger slice of onion on top of my burger!

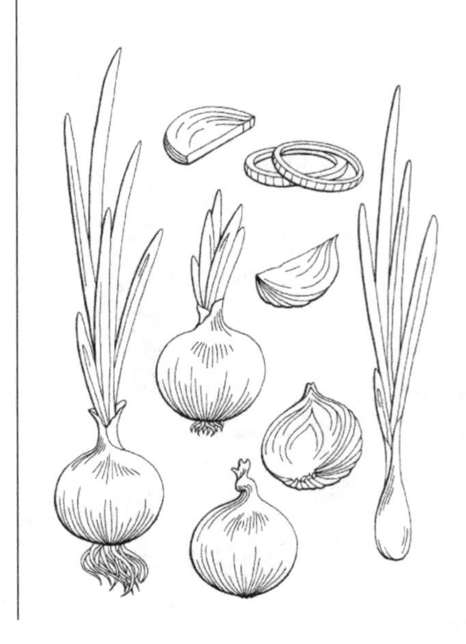

SPAGHETTI SQUASH

Spaghetti squash works well with a keto diet as a perfect replacement for wheat spaghetti noodles and is low in carbohydrates.

It bears a similar taste to traditional spaghetti noodles, and lends itself beautifully to a sumptuous dish when topped with marinara or spaghetti sauce.

Spaghetti squash originated in China, and I was surprised to learn that it was not introduced in the United States until 1936.

It boasts of B vitamins which are vital for optimal cellular function. Just like the avocado, spaghetti squash is also rich in folate, potassium, and high levels of beta carotene.

This member of the winter squash family is also a source of vitamin A and C which help prevent cell damage. Spaghetti squash is also high in omega-3 content which helps ward off heart disease by preventing inflammation in the body, and omega-6 fatty acids that aid in brain function.

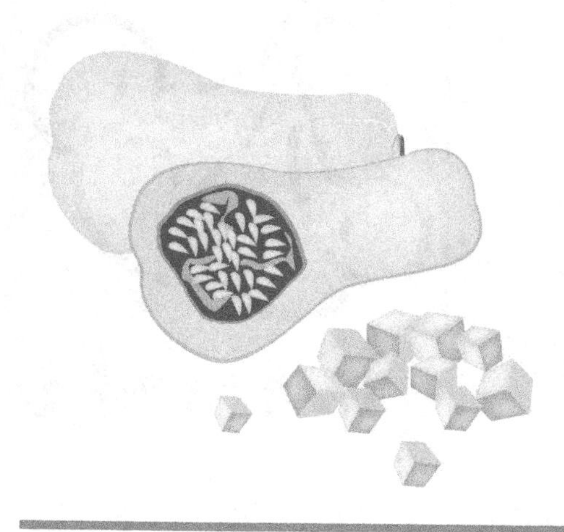

CRUCIFEROUS VEGETABLES

These amazing vegetables are packed with healthy nutrition and loaded with phytonutrients and antioxidants.

Cruciferous vegetables are a part of the cabbage family and consist of broccoli, cauliflower, kale, collards greens, Brussels sprouts, cabbage, bok choy, arugula, radishes, turnips, mustard greens, and watercress.

These vegetables are the stars in fiber, vitamins A and C, and folic acid. Cruciferous vegetables are rich in photochemical such as sulforaphane, which helps prevent cell damage by detoxifying carcinogens.

A study done in 1996[6] and posted in the journal *Cancer, Epidemiology, Biomarkers & Prevention*, stated that consuming cruciferous vegetables lowered risk of cancer.

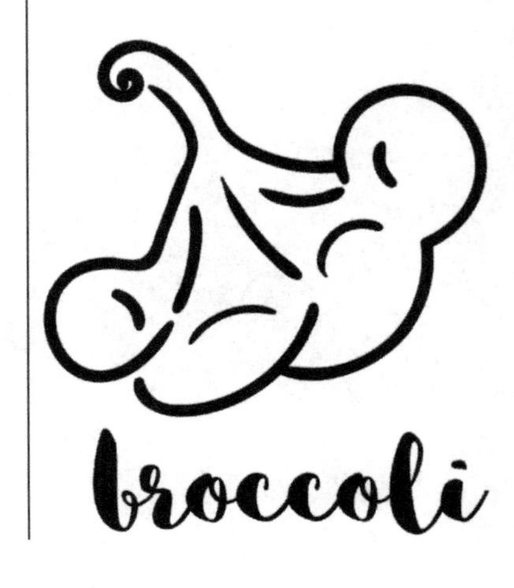

ASPARAGUS

The birthplace of asparagus was in Egypt over 2000 years ago and it was used for medicinal purposes. However, there is evidence that the Greeks began cultivating asparagus 500 years earlier than that!

In the United States, it can be traced back to the pilgrims.

Asparagus stands out from the crowd with its high concentration of heart healthy folate at a staggering 60%! Folate seems to be a superstar in many fruits and vegetables and asparagus leads the pack.

This nutrient protects fetus neural-tube birth defects causing spinal-bifida. Folate is a prescribed nutrient in neonatal vitamins for women who plan to get pregnant and those already pregnant.

Asparagus also provides vitamin E.

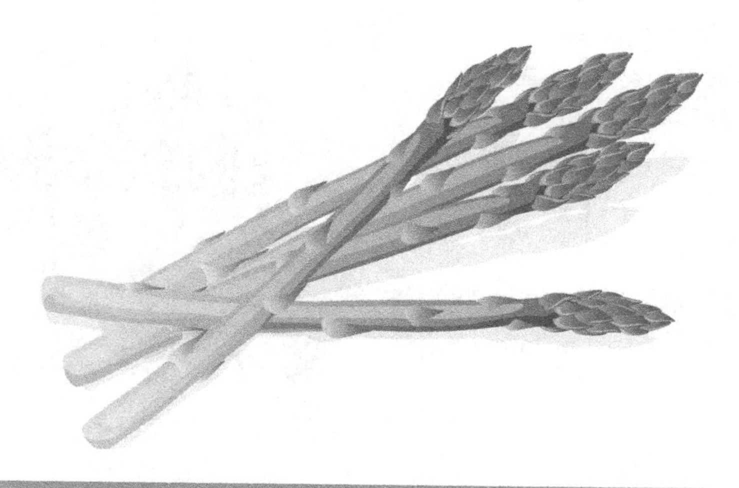

LEAFY GREENS

Leafy greens include all leaf lettuce and relatives' spinach, bok choy, and kale. All are loaded with vitamins A, C, E, and K.

This is one sure reason to indulge in a daily salad made up primarily of leafy greens, which have low carbs and are dense with water. A high fiber food, greens will help fill you up, especially when eaten at the beginning of a meal.

It is the high fiber in leafy greens that helps guard against constipation and can even lower cholesterol levels. They also have high levels of folic acid, lycopene, and alpha and beta-carotene, which help to guard against free-radical damage.

The lutein and zeaxanthin carotenoids protect the eye lens and macular region of the retina. Studies done in Sweden reported that consuming leafy greens reduced stomach cancer risk due to the bioflavonoid quercetin and its antioxidant and anti-inflammatory properties.

In researching leafy greens, I was amazed to discover a study at Rush University Medical Center[7] showed that leafy greens have an anti-aging effect due to vitamin K, folate, lutein, and beta-carotene presence. Cholesterol and triglyceride are enhanced in a positive way when leafy greens are consumed.

According to an Italian study, adding olive oil to your salad may enhance the benefits even more.

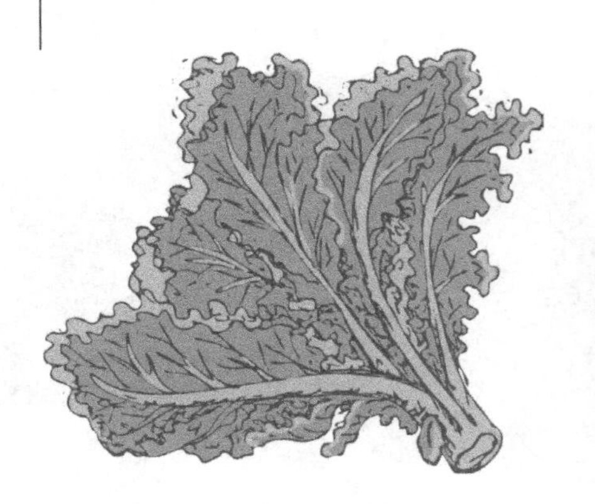

BERRIES

Berries might be small but don't let their size fool you. These little powerhouses are loaded with antioxidants ready to take up battle to ward off free radicals.

The power is in the purple, blue, and black colors of these little soldiers. Just like the grape and red wine, they are rich in dimethyl resveratrol.

Blueberries, raspberries, blackberries, and strawberries are perfect fruit for the keto diet as they are much lower in carbs than other fruits.

However, in the first four weeks of the keto diet, berries must be consumed in minimal amounts due to their fructose content.

Berries are also a source of magnesium, iron, and selenium.

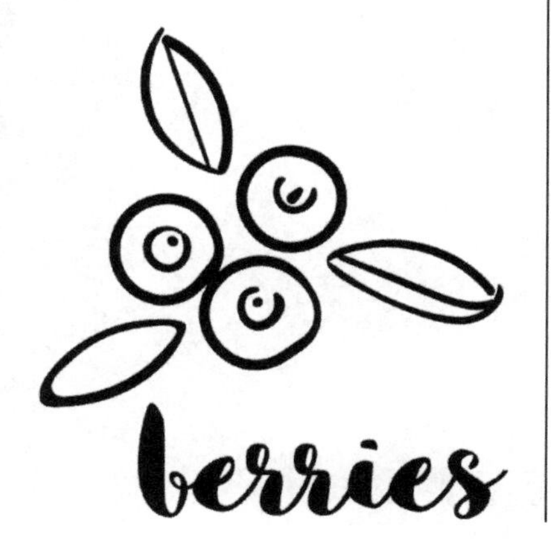

KETO FOR LIFE

28 Day Fat-Fueled
Approach To Weight Loss

PART THREE

RECIPES YOUR BODY WILL LOVE

"I will not start any sentence with the words 'I can't.' If I do, my mind will accept it as so, and then I won't be able to accomplish my goals. Instead I will tell myself, "I can," or "I will." In this way, success will come to me." *— Suzanne Somers*

Keto Recipes

Well, here we are where the excitement begins!

You finally made it to the keto recipes, and your challenge begins here. If you started here, I hope you will go back and read the beginning of the book, as there is so much valuable information that will help you understand how we got where we are today. Make this next chapter your own personal challenge to get the weight off once, and keep it off forever.

On the following pages you will find numerous recipes to help you in your quest for health and wellness. Please do not stress or be overwhelmed as you begin preparing the diet recipes. There are a lot of herbs and spices involved that enhance flavor to satisfy your taste buds.

If you are extremely busy and find it difficult to cook all the recipes, simply do what you can, but keep in mind that sugar and wheat are not your friends. If you don't eat red meat or don't like fish, just supplement with whatever protein you like.

Stay the course and use some of the tips throughout the book. Your quality of life is in your hands, so grab that shopping list and let's go!

— Barbara

Jumpstart Week 1 **Monday** Breakfast

Scrambled Eggs and Cheese with Sausage Patty

Serves One

Ingredients:

- 1 sausage patty
- 1 tablespoon olive oil
- 1 tablespoon butter
- 2 eggs
- One ounce shredded cheddar cheese
- Pepper to taste
- ¼ teaspoon parsley flakes

Directions:

1. Brown sausage patty in one tablespoon olive oil keeping the temperature low enough not to burn. Remove to breakfast plate.
2. Using a paper towel wipe skillet clean add one tablespoon butter and return to heat. Heat skillet to medium.
3. In small bowl whip two eggs and one ounce shredded cheddar cheese.
4. Add pepper and parsley flakes to egg mixture and add to skillet. Reduce heat to low. You may add additional herbs. Gently stir to prevent overcooking eggs.
5. Add scrambled eggs and cheese to breakfast plate with sausage patty.

NOTES

Record your thoughts starting Jumpstart Week 1:

Date:

Thoughts:

How I'm feeling now:

Weight:

Jumpstart Week 1 **Monday** Lunch

Sirloin Steak Salad

Serves Two

Ingredients:

- One 4 to 6-ounce sirloin steak
- 1 tablespoon avocado oil
- Salt and pepper to taste
- 3 cups of bagged salad greens
- 1 medium avocado sliced
- ¼ medium tomato peeled, sliced and seeded
- ¼ cup cucumber, sliced
- ½ cup mushrooms sliced
- 4 tablespoons Ken's low carb blue cheese dressing

**(This dressing is very thick, and you may wish to add 1 tablespoon olive oil to 2 tablespoons of Ken's.)*

Directions:

1. Heat small skillet and add avocado oil.
2. Add steak to hot skillet and brown to desired doneness.
3. Remove steak place on cutting board and slice diagonally.
4. Place salad greens on two large plates.
5. Slice all vegetables and spread on top of greens and add ½ sliced avocado to each plate.
6. Placed sliced steak on top of salad.
7. Dress with Ken's low carb ranch or blue cheese dressing.

You can control your future and you decide what actually becomes a reality. Focus on the outcome you want to achieve and allow yourself to be totally consumed by the joy of success!

— Barbara

Jumpstart Week 1 **Monday** Dinner

Baked Chicken Thighs with Cauliflower Mash

Serves Two

Ingredients:

- 2 pounds chicken thighs skin on and bone in
- ½ medium onion cut into large pieces
- 2 garlic cloves crushed
- ½ pound button mushrooms quartered
- ¼ cup olive oil
- ¼ cup chicken stock
- Dash basil
- Dash thyme
- Sea salt to taste

Directions: Chicken Thighs

1. Heat oven to 350 degrees.
2. Cut up onion and quarter mushrooms and place in medium sized shallow baking dish.
3. In a small bowl mix olive oil and chicken stock with garlic, basil, and thyme.
4. Place chicken in oven dish on top of onions and mushrooms.
5. Add olive oil and chicken stock mixture over the chicken.
6. Add salt and pepper.
7. Place in oven and bake uncovered for one hour.

Directions: Cauliflower Mash

1. ½ large cauliflower cut into florets.
2. Bring water to boil, reduce heat to medium, place cauliflower in a steamer basket over boiling water and cover.
3. Allow cauliflower to steam for 10 minutes.
4. Remove from heat drain and mash with potato masher or place in blender.
5. Add salt and pepper to taste (add one crushed garlic clove if you wish).

**Do not place cauliflower directly in water as it will become mushy.*

Jumpstart Week 1 **Tuesday** Breakfast

Poached Eggs with Avocado and Salsa

Serves One or Two

Ingredients:

- 2 medium to large eggs
- One avocado
- 2 tablespoon Chi-Chi's Salsa

Directions:

1. Poach eggs in boiling water or egg poaching pan. Break eggs open and place one at a time in a small bowl before adding to water. Carefully slide the eggs from the bowl into the simmering water. Using a large spoon shape the egg whites around the yolk. Cook eggs for 2 minutes for soft and about 4 minutes to fully cook.
2. Slice one avocado lengthwise into equal halves remove seed, peel and place on plate.
3. Lift eggs with slotted spoon and fill each half avocado with poached egg.
4. Scoop one tablespoon salsa on top of eggs.

Jumpstart Week 1 **Tuesday** Lunch

Tuna Fish Salad

Serves One

Ingredients:

- One 3 ounces can tuna fish oil or water packed
- One tablespoon chopped celery
- One tablespoon chopped onion
- 2 tablespoon Hellman's Mayonnaise
- One cup bagged salad greens
- One cup mixed vegetables of your choice
- One tablespoon olive oil or avocado oil
- Salt and pepper to taste

Directions:

1. Mix tuna, Mayonnaise, celery, and onion together.
2. Place salad greens and cut up vegetables on large plate.
3. Drizzle salad with either one tablespoon olive oil or avocado oil.
4. Scoop a mound of tuna mixture onto salad.

Jumpstart Week 1 **Tuesday** Dinner

Grilled Rosemary Lamb Chops with Green Peas and Salad

Serves Two

Ingredients:

- ½ cup frozen green peas
- Four 3 to 4-ounce lamb chops fat untrimmed
- 2 teaspoons olive oil
- 1 teaspoon crushed rosemary
- 1 garlic clove crushed
- Sea salt and ground black pepper to taste

Directions:

1. Combine olive oil, rosemary, and garlic in small sauce dish and rub both sides of lamb chops with the mixture.
2. Add a pinch of sea salt and ground black pepper to both sides of lamb chops.
3. Let lamb chops marinate and prepare salad.
4. Place lamb chops on hot grill and cook to desired doneness.
5. Microwave peas and season to taste.

Salad:

1. 1 cup bagged lettuce
2. ½ cup mixed vegetables of your choice
3. 2 tablespoons Ken's low carb ranch or blue cheese dressing

(This dressing is very thick, and you may wish to add one tablespoon olive oil to 2 tablespoons of Ken's.)

Jumpstart Week 1 **Wednesday** Breakfast

Old Fashion Deviled Eggs, Bacon and Spinach

Serves One

Ingredients:

- 2 large hard boiled eggs
- 2 strips bacon
- Handful baby spinach
- 1 tablespoon Hellman's Mayonnaise
- ¼ teaspoon Dijon mustard
- Salt and pepper to taste
- Dash paprika

Directions:

1. Place eggs in medium saucepan and add enough water to cover eggs. Bring to boil and cover. Reduce heat to low and cook eggs for approximately 10 minutes. Once done run cold water over eggs, and allow eggs to cool.
2. Cook bacon and place on plate.
3. Drain off most bacon fat and stir-fry spinach and add to plate.
4. Peel eggs and cut lengthwise and remove yolks to a small bowl.
5. Place empty egg white on top of spinach
6. Mash egg yolks with fork and blend with mayonnaise and mustard.
7. Place egg yolk mixture back in egg white and sprinkle with paprika.

(You may prepare eggs the night before to save time in the morning, or purchase pre-boiled eggs.)

Jumpstart Week 1 **Wednesday** Lunch

Shrimp Stuffed Avocado with Salad

Serves One

Ingredients:

- One 3.5 ounces canned medium shrimp
- One medium avocado
- 2 tablespoon Hellmann's Mayonnaise
- 1 teaspoon chopped fresh or dried chives
- Pinch of black pepper
- Dash of turmeric (optional)

Directions:

1. Open can drain and chop shrimp and place in medium bowl.
2. Add mayonnaise, chives, black pepper, and turmeric to shrimp and mix well.
3. Cut avocado in half lengthwise and remove pit first and then remove peel, using thumb and forefinger.
4. Place avocado halves on plate and fill with shrimp.
5. Add a dash of paprika.

Salad:

1. 1 cup bagged lettuce
2. ½ cup mixed vegetables of your choice
3. 2 tablespoons Ken's low carb ranch or blue cheese dressing

(This dressing is very thick, and you may wish to add one tablespoon olive oil to 2 tablespoons of Ken's.)

Jumpstart Week 1 **Wednesday** Dinner

Roasted Chicken with Broccoli and Salad

Serves One or Two

Ingredients:

- 1 rotisserie roasted chicken from Sam's Club, Whole Foods,or your local supermarket. (Save half for next day lunch.)
- 1 cup broccoli (fresh or frozen)
- One ounce shredded cheddar cheese

Directions:

1. Slice chicken to desired amount and place on plate.
2. Place broccoli in microwave dish and cook.
3. Add cheddar cheese to broccoli and melt. Place on dinner plate with chicken.

See Salad Ingredients and Directions on Page 135

Jumpstart Week 1 **Thursday** Breakfast

Smoked Salmon Cream Cheese and Eggs

Serves One

Ingredients:

- Divide 3 ounces smoked salmon into 4 strips
- One lemon wedge
- ¼ cup full fat cream cheese
- 1 teaspoon dried dill
- Ground black pepper
- One or two eggs

Directions:

1. Place salmon strips on large plate and squeeze lemon on top (optional).
2. Sprinkle dried dill and ground pepper over salmon strips.
3. Divide cream cheese and place on salmon strips and roll up.
4. Cook eggs any way desired, add to plate (You may eliminate eggs and add more salmon if you choose.)

Jumpstart Week 1 **Thursday** Lunch

Chicken Salad Stuffed Tomato

Serves One

Ingredients:

- One cup cooked chicken, white or dark meat, cut into bite-size pieces (Substitute chicken for tuna fish if you wish.)
- One medium tomato
- One tablespoon chopped onion
- Six halved grapes
- ¼ cup celery
- ¼ cup chopped walnuts
- ¼ cup Hellman's Mayonnaise
- ½ teaspoon Dijon mustard
- Salt and pepper to taste
- Dash paprika

Directions:

1. Place all ingredients in medium size bowl except mayonnaise and mustard.
2. In a small bowl stir mayonnaise and mustard together and spoon into chicken mixture.
3. Cut top off the tomato and cut vertically halfway down the center then rotate tomato and slice down center and press cut pieces open creating space for salad (You may remove seeds if you wish.)
4. Scoop chicken salad over tomato.
5. Salt and pepper to taste and dash of paprika.

Salad:

1. 1 cup bagged lettuce
2. ½ cup mixed vegetables of your choice
3. 2 tablespoons Ken's low carb ranch or blue cheese dressing

(This dressing is very thick, and you may wish to add one tablespoon olive oil to 2 tablespoons of Ken's.)

Jumpstart Week 1 **Thursday** Dinner

Baked Ham with Cheesy Mock Mashed Potato

Serves Two or Three

Ingredients:

- Small 2 to 3-pound ham pre-cooked or fresh
- ¼ teaspoon sage
- ½ teaspoon dried Rosemary
- Ground black pepper to taste

Directions:

1. Preheat oven to 350 degrees. (300 degrees if you are warming a precooked ham) Bake to time reference on the package.
2. Place ham in shallow baking dish and add ½ cup water to pan.
3. Sprinkle ham with sage, Rosemary, and pepper (Add any seasonings you wish).
4. Prepare Cheesy Mock Mashed Potato and Salad while ham is cooking.
5. Remove baked ham from oven and cool for ten minutes. Slice and place on plate.
6. Add a half cup mock mashed potato.

Cheesy Mock Mashed Potato

Ingredients:

- One head cauliflower
- 3 green onions chopped
- 1 garlic clove crushed
- 1 cup shredded cheddar cheese
- ¼ cup almond milk
- ½ cup grated parmesan cheese
- 2 tablespoons butter
- Salt and ground pepper to taste
- Preheat oven to 450 degrees

Directions:

1. Select a large stock pot and add 2 inches of water in the bottom.
2. Cut the bottom off cauliflower and break into very small florets.
3. Steam cauliflower for 8 to 10 minutes (It may take longer or divide into two parts if steamer is small).
4. Chop green onions using much of the stem.
5. Peel and crush garlic and add with onions to ½ cup shredded cheddar cheese.
6. Test cauliflower for doneness and add to large bowl.
7. Stir in cheese onion, garlic, and ¼ cup almond milk, mix well and place mixture in oven baking dish.
8. Melt butter in microwave dish and pour evenly over mock potatoes.
9. Place baking dish in oven and bake for approximately 10 minutes being careful not to burn.
10. Top with ½ cup grated cheese and salt and pepper to taste.

Jumpstart Week 1 **Friday** Breakfast

English Style Breakfast

Serves One

Ingredients:

- Two large eggs
- Two tablespoons butter or olive oil
- Two slices ham
- One link sausage
- One half cup mushrooms
- One plum tomato
- One half sliced avocado
- Salt and pepper to taste

Directions:

1. Melt butter in large skillet on low heat. Add ham sausage and mushrooms to skillet and sauté.
2. Slice tomato lengthwise and place in skillet cut side down in butter.
3. Push everything to side with spatula and add eggs.
4. Cook eggs to desired doneness and place on plate.
5. Add ham, mushrooms, sausage, tomato, and sliced avocado to plate.
6. Add salt and pepper to taste.

"Challenges are gifts that force us to search for a new center of gravity. Don't fight them. Just find a different way to stand."

— Oprah Winfrey

Jumpstart Week 1 **Friday** Lunch

Turkey Burgers and Guacamole

Serves Two

Ingredients:

- 3/4 pound ground turkey
- 2 tablespoon olive oil
- 2 garlic cloves crushed
- ½ cup chopped fresh cilantro
- ½ cup green onions chopped
- ½ teaspoon ground black pepper
- ½ teaspoon sea salt
- 1 cup fresh spinach

Directions

1. In a large mixing bowl add ground turkey, olive oil, crushed garlic, chopped cilantro, chopped green onions, salt, and pepper.
2. Mix all ingredients except spinach. Mash ingredients together completely to assure all are evenly distributed.
3. Divide the mixture evenly into four large patties and place on broiler pan or sided baking sheet.
4. Turn the broiler on high. Place pan under the broiler on the second level down from the top (about 6 inches).
5. Broil for 7 to 8 minutes per side being careful not to burn.
6. If you have a meat thermometer, the temperature should reach 165 degrees to assure doneness.
7. Prepare guacamole.

Guacamole

Ingredients:

- 2 ripe Avocados
- ½ small white onion
- 1 small tomato
- 1 garlic clove crushed
- 1 teaspoon lime juice
- Salt to taste
- ½ teaspoon red pepper flakes (optional)

Directions:

1. Cut avocados in half lengthwise, remove seed and peel using thumb and forefinger.
2. Place avocados in medium bowl and mash with a fork or potato masher. If you prefer large chunks, use a fork.
3. Add all the other ingredients and mix together.
4. Feel free to add any seasonings you like including hot sauce.
5. Prepare plate with one or two turkey patties, cup of spinach, and large mound of guacamole.

Jumpstart Week 1 **Friday** Dinner

Italian Sausage and Marinara Casserole with Vegetables

Serves Three to Four

Ingredients:

- One pound Italian Sausages
- 2 tablespoons olive oil
- 1 small white onion chopped
- ½ medium red pepper chopped and ½ medium green pepper chopped.
- 1 15.5 ounces jar of Roe's Marinara Sauce
- ½ teaspoon dried basil
- ½ teaspoon dried oregano
- ¼ cup grated parmesan cheese
- ½ teaspoon salt
- Ground black pepper to taste

Directions:

Add two tablespoons olive oil to skillet and brown sausages

1. Preheat oven to 350 degrees.
2. Place sausages in 9 x 13 baking dish.
3. Open Roe's Marinara Sauce and pour into hot skillet, stir in basil, oregano, salt, and pepper.
4. Layer sausages with onion, red and green peppers.
5. Pour Roe's Marinara Sauce and seasonings from skillet over sausages and top with chopped basil and ¼ cup grated parmesan cheese.
6. Bake in the oven for 45 minutes.

Jumpstart Week 1 **Saturday** Breakfast

Eggs Benedict with Hollandaise and Canadian Bacon

Serves One or Two

Ingredients

- 2 large eggs
- 2 pieces Canadian bacon
- ½ avocado
- 1 tablespoon lemon juice
- Ground pepper to taste
- Salt to taste

Directions:

1. Preheat oven to 350 degrees. Rub two ramekins with olive oil and place Canadian bacon rounds in ramekins and push to bottom creating a nest for eggs.
2. Break one egg into each ramekin and place in preheated oven and bake to the desired doneness.
3. Prepare hollandaise while eggs are baking.
4. Slice half avocado and place on plate.

Hollandaise Sauce

Ingredients:

- 2 egg yolks
- 1 tablespoon lemon juice
- Dash ground pepper
- Dash paprika

Directions:

1. Whisk egg yolks in small bowl.
2. Melt ¼ cup butter in the microwave.
3. Whisk lemon juice and pepper into egg yolks.
4. Slowly pour warm melted butter over egg yolks whisking constantly to prevent cooking yolks.
5. Remove poached eggs from oven and place on two plates. Drizzle hollandaise evenly over eggs and top with sprinkle of paprika.

Jumpstart Week 1 **Saturday** Lunch

Salmon Fillet and Tartar Sauce with Sautéed Asparagus and Salad

Serves Two

Prepare tartar sauce first

Easy Tartar Sauce

Ingredients:

- 2 tablespoons Hellman's Mayonnaise
- 2 tablespoons sour cream
- 1 teaspoon dried dill

Directions:

1. Mix all above ingredients together and place in fridge.

Salmon Fillet

Ingredients:

- ½ pound salmon (2 fillets)
- 2 teaspoons olive oil
- 1 teaspoon dried dill
- Salt to taste
- Ground pepper to taste
- Serve with tartar sauce

Directions:

1. Rub each salmon fillet with 1 teaspoons olive oil.
2. Sprinkle ½ teaspoon dried dill on each fillet.
3. Salt and pepper to taste.
4. Place salmon under the broiler and cook for 8 to 10 minutes.
5. Sauté asparagus while salmon is cooking.

Sautéed Asparagus

Ingredients:

- 2 tablespoons butter
- ½ pound asparagus
- Salt and pepper to taste
- Dash of garlic salt (optional)

Directions:

1. Heat large skillet to medium and melt butter. Add asparagus to skillet and add salt, pepper, and garlic salt to taste.
2. Sauté until desired doneness.
3. Place on large dinner plate with salmon and tartar sauce.

See Salad Ingredients and Directions on Page 135.

Jumpstart Week 1 **Saturday** Dinner

Lamb Burgers with Greek Salad

Serves Two

Ingredients:

- ½ pound ground lamb
- ½ small red onion chopped
- 1 garlic clove crushed
- ½ teaspoon ground cumin
- ¼ teaspoon turmeric (optional)
- ¼ cup feta cheese
- 1 tablespoon avocado or olive oil
- Salt and pepper to taste to taste

Directions:

1. Combine all above ingredients except avocado oil.
2. Divide mixture into two equal parts and shape into patties.
3. Add avocado oil to skillet and heat to medium.
4. Place lamb patties in pan and brown on both sides for approximately 5 minutes on each side.
5. Place on plate and serve with Greek Salad.

Greek Salad

Ingredients:

- ½ cucumber, sliced
- ½ medium tomato sliced
- ½ green pepper, sliced
- ½ onion, sliced
- ½ cup kalamata olives, pitted
- One teaspoon chopped parsley
- ½ cup feta cheese
- 6 tablespoons olive oil
- 2 tablespoons balsamic vinegar
- Salt and pepper to taste

Directions:

1. Mix all ingredients together in a large bowl and divide between two salad plates.

Jumpstart Week 1 **Sunday** Breakfast

Mushroom and Swiss Cheese Omelet

Serves Two

Ingredients:

- 2 tablespoon butter
- 2 ounces white button mushrooms
- 2 green onions with stems
- 1 clove garlic crushed
- ¼ teaspoon dried thyme
- 4 eggs
- ½ cup shredded Swiss cheese
- ¼ teaspoon dried parsley flakes
- Salt and pepper to taste
- 2 tablespoon Chi Chi's Salsa

Directions:

1. Place skillet on stove and add 1 tablespoon butter and heat to medium temperature.
2. Slice mushrooms and green onions and add to hot skillet.
3. Crush garlic and thyme; add to skillet and sauté until onions are translucent.
4. Remove from skillet and place above ingredients in small bowl.
5. In a larger bowl whip 4 eggs, cheese, and parsley.
6. Add mushroom, onions, and garlic to egg mixture and mix well.
7. Divide into two equal amounts.
8. Place 1 tablespoon butter to skillet. Sloping sides work best to manage the omelet. Lift the edges as it cooks to assure uniform doneness.
9. Top each omelet with a tablespoon Chi Chi's Salsa.

Jumpstart Week 1 **Sunday** Lunch

Sloppy Joes Stuffed Peppers

Serves Two

Ingredients:

- Preheat oven to 350 degrees
- 2 red bell peppers
- 1 tablespoon butter
- 1 small white onion chopped
- ½ green bell pepper, chopped
- 1 tablespoon olive oil
- 1 pound ground beef
- 1 tablespoon Dijon mustard
- ¼ teaspoon red pepper flakes (optional
- 1 small can tomato paste (unsweetened)
- 1-14 ounce canned chopped tomatoes (unsweetened)
- Salt and pepper to taste

Directions:

1. Wash, remove stems, cut red peppers in two and remove seeds and place in baking dish. Place in hot oven and bake for 20 minutes while preparing sloppy Joe mixture.
2. Melt 1 tablespoon butter in skillet; add onion, green pepper and sauté.
3. Add olive oil and ground beef to skillet and brown.
4. Add Dijon mustard, red pepper flakes, and stir into beef mixture.
5. Add tomato paste and chopped tomatoes and continue cooking until bubbly.
6. Remove red peppers from oven, place on plate, and fill with Sloppy Joe mixture.

Jumpstart Week 1 **Sunday** Dinner

Pork Chops with Almond Green Beans and Salad

Serves Two

**Prepare salad just before cooking pork chops*

See Salad Ingredients and Directions on Page 135.

Ingredients:

- 2 large bone in well-marbled pork chops
- 1/3 cup coconut flour
- 1 teaspoon Himalayan Sea Salt
- 1 teaspoon ground black pepper
- Garlic salt to taste
- 1 ½ tablespoons butter
- 2 teaspoons olive oil for rubbing pork chops

Directions:

1. Place all ingredients except butter in a gallon sized zip-lock bag.
2. Rub pork chops with olive oil and place individually into zip-lock bag and shake well to coat.
3. Place 1 1/2 tablespoons butter in skillet and heat slowly to medium temperature to prevent burning. Add pork chops to skillet and pan fry for 5 minutes per side until the desired doneness. You may broil pork chops if you wish.
4. While pork chops are cooking prepare green beans and mushrooms.

Almond Green Beans and Mushrooms

Ingredients:

- One small bag frozen green beans
- 1 small can sliced mushrooms
- ¼ cup slivered almonds
- Salt to taste
- Pepper to taste

Directions:

1. Open canned mushrooms and place in microwave safe dish with liquid (do not drain liquid).
2. Place green beans in with mushrooms and microwave according to package directions.
3. Drain off liquid and add almonds.
4. Add a tablespoon of butter and stir into green beans and mushrooms to melt.
5. Place green beans with pork chops on dinner plate and serve with salad.

Jumpstart Week 2 **Monday** Breakfast

No Crust Quiche with Cheddar Cheese and Spinach

Serves Four

Ingredients:

- 4 large eggs
- ½ cup heavy cream
- 1 small package frozen spinach
- 1 cup shredded cheddar cheese
- 3 strips cook crumbled bacon
- Salt and pepper to taste

Directions:

1. Preheat oven to 350 degrees.
2. Thaw and drain spinach pat dry with paper towel.
3. Grease quiche dish or 9-inch pie plate.
4. Brown bacon strips in skillet, cool and crumble.
5. In a large bowl whip eggs and heavy cream.
6. Add salt and pepper.
7. Add bacon, spinach, and cheese.
8. Mix well and pour into quiche dish and bake.
9. Bake for 35 to 40 minutes (To test doneness insert knife in center. Knife should come out clean when done.)

NOTES

Record your thoughts starting Jumpstart Week 2:

Date:

Thoughts:

How I'm feeling now:

Weight:

Jumpstart Week 2 **Monday** Lunch

Niçoise Salad with Tuna and Avocado

Serves Two

Ingredients:

- One 5 ounces can tuna drained
- 1 avocado
- 2 hardboiled eggs
- 4 ounces green beans
- 1 medium tomato halved and sliced lengthwise
- 1 head Boston lettuce washed and dried
- 1 small red onion
- ¼ cup black olives pitted (you may substitute green olives)
- Salt and ground black pepper

Directions:

1. Place eggs in medium saucepan and add enough water to cover eggs. Bring to boil and cover. Reduce heat to low and cook eggs for approximately 10 minutes. Once done run cold water over eggs.
2. Microwave or steam green beans.
3. Prepare two large plates with equal halves lettuce torn into bite-size pieces.
4. Slice avocado in half lengthwise and remove pit, then peel and slice one half for each plate.
5. Divide green beans equally between two plates.
6. Peel onion and cut into thin slices dividing equally.
7. Peel eggs and slice each egg into four wedges and place on plates.
8. Add black olives.

Dressing

- 2 tablespoons Ken's low carb vinaigrette, ranch or blue cheese per plate (if you want to stretch the dressing add a tablespoon of olive oil)
- Salt and Pepper to taste

Jumpstart Week 2 **Monday** Dinner

Slow Cooker Corned Beef and Sauerkraut with Salad

Serves Four

Ingredients:

- 4-pound corned beef brisket with seasoning pack
- 1 bag sauerkraut (usually found in deli section of supermarket)

Directions:

1. Set slow cooker temperature on low and add corned beef brisket fat side up, sprinkle seasonings over brisket and cook for 4 hours.
2. Drain juice from sauerkraut and discard.
3. Do not add salt as briskets can be very salty.
4. Add drained sauerkraut and dump on top of brisket
5. (Briskets typically have high water content so it is not necessary to add more liquid, however, add a small amount of water if you see brisket looks dry).
6. Cover and continue cooking for 2 more hours
7. (If you must be gone all day, it is okay to add the sauerkraut to the brisket.)

Salad:

1. 1 cup bagged lettuce
2. ½ cup mixed vegetables of your choice
3. 2 tablespoons Ken's low carb ranch or blue cheese dressing

(This dressing is very thick, and you may wish to add one tablespoon olive oil to 2 tablespoons of Ken's.)

Jumpstart Week 2 **Tuesday** Breakfast

Salmon and Cream Cheese Rollups with Two Eggs

Serves One

Ingredients:

- 4 ounces smoked salmon
- ¼ cup full-fat cream cheese
- ½ teaspoon dried dill
- 1 teaspoon capers
- 1 tablespoon chopped onion
- Ground pepper to taste

Directions

1. Divide smoked salmon into 4 strips.
2. Mix cream cheese and dill together and spread equal amounts on salmon strips.
3. Sprinkle capers and onion over salmon.
4. Add ground pepper to taste.
5. Prepare one or two eggs any way you like them and add to plate with salmon.

Jumpstart Week 2 **Tuesday** Lunch

Leftover Corned Beef and Sauerkraut with Avocado

Serves Two

Directions:

1. Heat desired amount of corned beef and sauerkraut in the microwave for approximately 2 minutes.
2. Divide one avocado and remove pit and peel.
3. Place half avocado on each plate and add one tablespoon Hellman's Mayonnaise to each half.

Jumpstart Week 2 **Tuesday** Dinner

Roasted Rack of Lamb with Asparagus and Salad

Serves Two

Ingredients:

- 1 ½ pound lamb rack with ribs exposed
- 2 tablespoons olive oil
- 2 cloves garlic crushed
- 1 teaspoon chopped thyme
- 1 teaspoon chopped rosemary
- Ground black pepper to taste
- Himalayan pink salt to taste

Directions:

1. Set oven temperature at 450 degrees.
2. Place rack on baking sheet with sides to contain drippings.
3. Place lamb with ribs up and wrap rib ends with foil to prevent burning.
4. Rub rack of lamb thoroughly with olive oil.
5. Add crushed garlic and rub into lamb.
6. Sprinkle thyme and rosemary over rack.
7. Add salt and pepper to taste.
8. Place in oven and bake for 15 minutes at 450 degrees.
9. Lower heat to 325 degrees for another 15 minutes.
10. Test meat for desired doneness.
11. Remove from oven and allow to set for 10 minutes.
12. Remove foil from legs, divide and plate.

**Prepare asparagus and salad while lamb is cooking*

Sauteed Asparagus

Directions:

1. ½ pound asparagus.
2. Add ¼ cup olive oil to large skillet and add asparagus.
3. Add salt and pepper to taste and dash of garlic salt if desired.
4. Sauté until desired doneness.
5. Place on large dinner plate with lamb.

Salad:

1. 1 cup bagged lettuce
2. ½ cup mixed vegetables of your choice
3. 2 tablespoons Ken's low carb ranch or blue cheese dressing

(This dressing is very thick, and you may wish to add one tablespoon olive oil to 2 tablespoons of Ken's.)

Jumpstart Week 2 **Wednesday** Breakfast

Pancakes with Berries and Whipped Cream

Serves Two

Ingredients:

- 4-ounce carton extra thick whipping cream
- 4 drops liquid stevia (2 for whipped cream and 2 for berries)
- ¼ teaspoon vanilla
- 1/3 cup Philadelphia brand cream cheese. Use the creamy style that comes in a tub.
- 1 cup almond flour
- 1 teaspoon baking soda
- Dash of ground nutmeg
- ¼ teaspoon cinnamon
- 4 eggs
- ½ cup almond milk (if batter is too thick add more almond milk slowly to reach desired consistency)
- 1 teaspoon vanilla
- 3 to 4 tablespoons butter for griddle and pancakes

Directions:

1. ½ cup fresh or frozen raspberries or blueberries.
2. Mash berries slightly to create some juice. You may add 2 drop of stevia to sweeten.
3. Place whipping cream and in small bowl and whip until thick and fluffy and add 2 drops liquid stevia and vanilla.
4. Place whipped cream in the refrigerator while preparing pancakes.
5. Preheat griddle to medium high.
6. In a medium bowl combine almond flour, baking soda, nutmeg, and cinnamon.
7. In a small bowl whisk or beat eggs, add cream cheese, almond milk, and vanilla. Continue whisking until well blended.
8. Add egg mixture to flour mixture and whisk to combine.
9. Pour batter onto griddle for each pancake (you may make 4 large pancakes if you choose).
10. You may continue cooking leftover batter and place individually in quart size bags and freeze. (Do not put two pancakes in one bag unless you wrap them first in saran wrap to prevent sticking together).
11. Once pancakes are ready, place on plate and top with butter, heavy whipping cream, and berries or sugar-free syrup.

Jumpstart Week 2 **Wednesday** Lunch

Hamburger Salad with Cheese

Serves One

Ingredients:

- One cup salad greens
- One cup mixed vegetables
- ¼ pound hamburger (not lean)
- Salt and pepper to taste
- 1-ounce cheddar or cheese of your choice

Directions:

1. Place salad greens and vegetables on large plate.
2. Add two tablespoons Ken's low carb dressing (you may also add 1 tablespoon olive oil to dressing).
3. Grill or broil hamburger and melt cheese on top if you wish or add cheese to salad.
4. Place burger on top of salad and add dressing.

"The ultimate measure of a man is not where he stands in moments of comfort and convenience, but where he stands at times of challenge and controversy."
— Martin Luther King, Jr.

Jumpstart Week 2 **Wednesday** Dinner

Stir-fry Shrimp with Vegetables and Caprese Salad

Serves Two

Ingredients:

- One pound thawed medium shrimp, tails removed, deveined
- One small red onion chopped
- 2 garlic cloves crushed
- 1 bunch broccoli cut into small florets
- ¼ pound white button or shitake mushrooms sliced
- 2 tablespoons soy sauce
- 2 tablespoon sesame oil
- ½ cup chicken stock
- 1 bag pre-washed baby spinach
- Salt and pepper to taste

Directions:

1. Mix together chicken stock, soy sauce, and sesame oil.
2. Heat wok to medium high heat, add one tablespoon olive oil and sauté shrimp until partially done. Remove from wok and set aside.
3. Add balance of olive oil and sauté broccoli, onion and garlic until broccoli florets are tender (2 or 3 minutes).
4. Add mushrooms and shrimp to wok and continue sautéing.
5. Stir and pour chicken stock mixture over shrimp and vegetables and continue stirring and cooking until shrimp are cooked (about 3 minutes).
6. Divide spinach equally between two dinner plates.
7. Divide shrimp stir-fry and place half on top of spinach.
8. Top with ground black pepper and salt to taste.

Caprese Salad **Serves Two**

Ingredients:

- ½ medium tomato
- ½ pound fresh mozzarella cheese
- ¼ cup fresh basil leaves
- ¼ cup extra virgin olive oil
- 2 teaspoons balsamic vinaigrette
- Himalayan pink salt to taste
- Ground black pepper to taste

Directions:

1. On two salad plates alternate 2 thin slices of tomato and two slices mozzarella cheese.
2. Garnish with basil leaves.
3. Divide olive oil and drizzle half on each plate.
4. Drizzle 1 teaspoon balsamic vinegar on each plate.
5. Add salt and pepper to taste.

Jumpstart Week 2 **Thursday** Breakfast

Bacon and Cheese Omelet with Avocado

Serves One

Ingredients:

- 4 slices bacon
- 2 large eggs
- 1 tablespoon butter
- 1 ounce shredded cheddar, provolone or cheese of your choice
- ½ avocado
- 1 tablespoon Hellman's Mayonnaise

Directions:

1. Brown bacon in skillet and set aside.
2. Wipe skillet clean and heat to medium.
3. Add butter and melt.
4. Whisk eggs and add to skillet.
5. Reduce heat to low.
6. When eggs are nearly cooked through, flip over.
7. Spread cheese out on eggs and fold omelet in two.
8. Wait 30 seconds and flip omelet over and cook another 30 seconds.
9. Cut avocado in half and remove pit and peel.
10. Place omelet and bacon on large plate with half avocado and mayo.

NOTES:

Thoughts so far:

Jumpstart Week 2 **Thursday** Lunch

Cobb Salad

Serves Two

Ingredients:

- 2 peeled hard boiled eggs
- 4 slices bacon
- 1 bag prewashed romaine lettuce
- 1 cup chopped watercress (remove tough stems)
- 2 cups cooked chicken diced (Purdue has cooked chicken pieces in a bag, and it is a great product)
- 1 avocado halved, peeled, and diced with seed removed
- 1 medium tomato, chopped
- ¼ pound crumbled blue or Roquefort cheese

Directions:

1. Divide lettuce and place on two large plates.
2. Dice Chicken and place on plate.
3. Crumble bacon and add half to each plate.
4. Add half chopped tomato and diced avocado to each plate.
5. Crumble Roquefort cheese and arrange on plates.
6. Add chopped watercress to each plate.

Dressing

2 tablespoons Ken's low carb ranch, blue cheese, or Italian dressing. You may add 2 tablespoons olive oil to mix with Ken's.

Jumpstart Week 2 **Thursday** Dinner

Parmesan Crusted Chicken with Baked Zucchini

Serves Two

Ingredients:

- Four chicken thighs bone in and skin on
- ¼ cup olive oil
- ½ cup grated parmesan cheese
- 1 tablespoons butter
- Himalayan pink salt to taste
- Ground black pepper to taste

Directions:

1. Preheat oven to 375 degrees.
2. Place chicken thighs on plate and rub with olive oil.
3. Cover thighs evenly with grated parmesan cheese.
4. Press parmesan cheese into thighs.
5. Use 1 tablespoon butter, grease oven dish.
6. Place chicken thighs in a 7 x 11 or 8 x 8 oven dish.
7. Bake chicken for 40 minutes.

Parmesan Cheddar Baked Zucchini

Serves Two

Ingredients:

- 4 small zucchini
- 1 tablespoon olive oil
- 1 clove garlic crushed
- 1 teaspoon dried thyme
- 2 eggs
- 1/3 cup sour cream
- ½ cup shredded cheddar cheese
- ¼ cup shredded parmesan cheese
- Himalayan pink salt to taste
- Ground black pepper to taste

Directions:

8. Preheat oven to 375 degrees.
9. Grease 8 x 12 oven dish with olive oil.
10. Slice zucchini into ¼ inch slices and spread out in baking dish.
11. In a medium bowl whisk eggs, sour cream, garlic, and thyme.
12. Pour mixture over zucchini and bake for 40 minutes.

(If you are preparing this dish to serve with the chicken recipe above, prepare it first, as it will be baking for the same period of time and temperature as chicken)

See Salad Ingredients and Directions on Page 135.

Jumpstart Week 2 **Friday** Breakfast

Bacon and Eggs with Cream Cheese

Serves One

Ingredients:

- 3 slices bacon
- 2 eggs
- 1 tablespoon butter
- Salt and pepper to taste
- One ounce cream cheese

Directions:

1. Place 3 slices bacon in skillet and brown
2. Place bacon on plate
3. Drain bacon fat and wipe pan clean with paper towel
4. (You may use bacon fat to cook eggs if you wish)
5. Melt 1 tablespoon butter in skillet and prepare eggs
6. (You may prepare eggs any way you like them)
7. Place eggs, and cream cheese on plate with bacon

"It is our choices... that show what we really are, far more than out abilities."
— J.K. Rowling

Jumpstart Week 2 **Friday** Lunch

Chicken Salad and Bacon Wraps

Serves Two

Ingredients:

- One cup precooked chicken (Perdue has a 9-ounce bag of precooked chicken in what they call "short strips" and is perfect for this salad)
- 4 slices bacon
- ¼ cup mayonnaise
- ¼ cup sour cream
- 1 teaspoon dried dill
- 1 green onion
- 1 garlic clove crushed
- ½ tomato
- 1 avocado halved, pitted and peeled
- ½ cup feta cheese
- 1 head butter lettuce

Directions:

1. Place bacon strips in skillet and brown until crispy. Place on paper towel and set aside.
2. Wash and dry butter lettuce. Place on plate and create two nests for salad wraps. (You may use as much of the butter lettuce as you want.)
3. Mix together mayonnaise, sour cream, dried dill, crushed garlic, and chopped green onion in a bowl. Whisk to blend ingredients and set aside.
4. Divide chicken and place in each lettuce nest.
5. Crumble bacon and place on top of chicken.
6. Chop or slice tomato placing half on each wrap.
7. Cut avocado in half, pit, and peel. Slice avocado into strips and place half on each wrap.
8. Divide mayonnaise dressing and place half on each lettuce wrap.

Jumpstart Week 2 **Friday** Dinner

Herbed Pork Chops and Marsala Wine with Creamed Spinach

Serves Two

Ingredients:

- ¼ cup almond flour
- ½ teaspoon dried oregano
- ½ teaspoon garlic powder
- 2 large bone in pork chops
- 2 tablespoons butter
- ¼ cup olive oil
- 1 cup sliced fresh mushrooms
- 1 clove garlic crushed
- ¼ cup Marsala wine
- ¼ cup chicken stock

Directions:

1. Rub pork chops with 1 tablespoon olive oil.
2. Place almond flour, oregano, and garlic powder in gallon size Ziploc bag. Shake bag well to mix ingredients. Add pork chops one at a time and shake bag to coat pork chops completely.
3. Heat large skillet to medium and melt butter. Place pork chops in skillet and brown on both sides for about 10 minutes. Add mushrooms and crushed garlic and cook 5 minutes.
4. Add wine and chicken stock to skillet, cover and continue cooking

Creamed Spinach

Ingredients:

- 2 tablespoons butter
- 2 garlic cloves peeled and crushed
- ¼ cup chopped onion
- 1/3 cup heavy whipping cream
- ¼ teaspoon Himalayan pink salt
- ¼ teaspoon pepper
- 2 ounces shredded mozzarella cheese

Directions:

1. Heat large skillet to medium and melt butter.
2. Add garlic and onions to skillet and sauté.
3. Pour in heavy cream and add salt and pepper.
4. Stir in mozzarella cheese.
5. Reduce heat to low and continue stirring mixture until cheese is melted.
6. Add 8 ounces bagged prewashed spinach and stir into cream mixture.

See Salad Ingredients and Directions on Page 135.

Jumpstart Week 2 **Saturday** Breakfast

Omelet with Mozzarella Cheese and Avocado

Serves One

Ingredients:

- 3 eggs
- 1 ounce shredded mozzarella
- ½ avocado pitted and peeled
- ¼ medium tomato chopped
- 1 green onion chopped
- 1 tablespoon butter
- 1 tablespoon full fat sour cream
- 1 tablespoon Chi Chi's Salsa
- Salt and pepper to taste

Directions:

1. Preheat skillet to medium and add butter.
2. Whisk 3 eggs together in medium sized bowl.
3. Add salt and pepper to eggs and pour eggs into skillet.
4. Cook one side until nearly cooked through.
5. Flip cooked eggs over and add tomato and green onion.
6. Add mozzarella cheese and fold omelet over.
7. Cook one side about 30 seconds and flip over and cook for another 30 seconds.
8. Add to large plate and top with sour cream and Chi Chi's Salsa.
9. Slice avocado and place on plate with omelet.

Jumpstart Week 2 **Saturday** Lunch

Deli Ham or Turkey Romaine Lettuce Wrap

Serves Two

Ingredients:

- 1 head romaine lettuce
- ½ chopped tomato
- 1 avocado halved, pitted and peeled
- 2 tablespoons Hellman's mayonnaise
- 2 teaspoons spicy mustard (You may use any mustard)

Directions:

1. Wash and dry lettuce.
2. Place two or three leaves on each plate.
3. Mix mayonnaise and spicy mustard together in small bowl and spread equal amounts on each wrap.
4. Place deli meat, tomato, and avocado on top of mayo mixture.
5. Roll up lettuce folding one end over to hold filling.

"Change starts and ends with you. When you accept the challenge and do the work, the results rest in your hands."
— Barbara

Jumpstart Week 2 **Saturday** Dinner

Keto Crab Cakes with Stir-fry Spinach and Green Salad

Serves Two

Ingredients:

- One 8 ounce can crabmeat drained
- ¼ cup almond flour
- 2 tablespoon Hellman's Mayonnaise
- 1 egg
- ¼ teaspoon dried dill
- ¼ cup chopped white onion
- ½ teaspoon dried mustard
- ¼ teaspoon dried red pepper salt (optional)
- ¼ teaspoon celery salt
- ¼ teaspoon black pepper
- ¼ teaspoon Himalayan pink salt
- 3 tablespoons butter (You may use olive oil if you wish)

Directions:

1. In a medium-sized bowl, whisk egg well and add almond flour and mayo and whisk into egg.
2. Add dill, onion, mustard, red pepper, celery salt, black pepper, and Himalayan salt to egg mixture and whisk well.
3. Add crab meat to mixture and mix in well.
4. Form crab mixture into two or four patties.
5. Add 2 tablespoons butter to skillet and heat to medium high.
6. Using a spatula carefully place crab cakes in skillet.
7. Cook for up to five minutes on each side depending on size of cakes.
8. Place crab cakes on two large plates.

Stir-fry Spinach **Serves Two**

Ingredients:

- 1 tablespoon butter
- 1 garlic clove minced
- 2 bags pre-washed spinach (approximately 8 ounces)
- 1 tablespoon grated parmesan cheese
- Salt and pepper to taste

Directions:

1. Heat skillet to medium and add one tablespoon of butter. Add minced garlic to skillet and sauté for one minute.
2. Add baby spinach to skillet and sauté for one or two minutes until spinach is wilted.
3. Sprinkle one tablespoon grated Parmesan cheese over cooked spinach.
4. Place spinach on plate and add salt and pepper to taste.

Jumpstart Week 2 **Sunday** Breakfast

Denver Omelet with Sour Cream and Avocado

Serves Two

Ingredients:

- 1 tablespoon butter
- 2 green onions with stems
- ¼ red bell pepper, chopped
- ¼ green bell pepper, chopped
- 1 garlic clove crushed
- 4 eggs whisked
- ¼ cup diced cooked ham
- ½ cup shredded cheddar cheese
- Himalayan pink salt and ground black pepper to taste

Directions:

1. Heat skillet or omelet pan to medium and melt one tablespoon butter.
2. Add thinly sliced green onion including part of stem, add garlic, chopped red bell pepper, and diced ham.
3. Sauté for 3 or 4 minutes until vegetables are cooked, and ham is heated through.
4. In a medium bowl whisk eggs until yolk and white are well blended. Add cooked vegetables and ham to eggs.
5. Add one tablespoon butter and return pan to medium heat.
6. Divide egg mixture into two parts and pour ½ mixture into skillet and cook nearly through.
7. Flip first omelet over and spread ½ shredded parmesan cheese over omelet and fold omelet over.
8. Continue cooking one folded side for about 30 seconds and flip to other side and 30 seconds.
9. Move to large plate and cook the second omelet.
10. When omelets are ready, add ½ sliced, pitted, and peeled avocado to each plate and top each omelet with one tablespoon sour cream.

Jumpstart Week 2 **Sunday** Lunch

Grilled Steak Salad with Blue Cheese and Kale

Serves Two

Ingredients:

- ½ pound sirloin or steak of your choice
- Garlic salt to taste
- ½ teaspoon Montreal Steak Seasoning
- Himalayan pink salt to taste
- Ground black pepper to taste
- One tablespoon olive oil
- ½ cup crumbled blue cheese

Directions:

1. Pre-heat grill or oven broiler.
2. Rub steak entirely with olive oil.
3. Sprinkle steak with garlic salt, Montreal Steak Seasoning, Himalayan salt, and ground pepper.
4. Place steak on hot grill or put in oven under broiler.
5. (You may pan fry steak if you choose)
6. Prepare salad while steak is cooking

Salad:

Directions:

1. Double salad recipe for two.
2. One cup kale.
3. ½ cup mixed vegetables
4. 2 tablespoons Ken's low carb dressing.
5. Place salad mixture on plate and divide ½ cup of blue cheese between two plates.
6. Add salad dressing to salads.
7. Slice steak when ready and divide between two salad plates.

Jumpstart Week 2 **Sunday** Dinner

Crockpot Lemon Chicken with Green Beans

Serves Four

Ingredients:

- One 3 pound Purdue chicken
- One teaspoon dried oregano
- Himalayan pink salt to taste
- Pepper to taste
- Two garlic cloves crushed
- 3 tablespoons butter
- 1/3 cup water
- One lemon ends removed and lemon sliced thin

Directions:

1. Heat Crockpot to medium.
2. Season chicken inside and out with salt, pepper, oregano, and garlic
3. Heat large skillet to medium high and melt butter.
4. Place seasoned chicken in skillet and brown on all sides.
5. Remove chicken and place in Crockpot.
6. Add water to skillet and scrape chicken dripping.
7. Add thinly sliced lemon to pan and cook for one minute and pour over browned chicken.
8. Using a long-handled fork, place two lemon slices inside chicken.
9. Place Crockpot cover over chicken and cook on low for eight hours.
10. Carve the chicken and pour sauce from Crockpot over chicken.
11. Place the desired amount of chicken on each plate. (Save one cup of leftover chicken for Monday's lunch.)

Green Beans with Parmesan and Garlic

Serves Two

Ingredients:

- ½ pound green beans
- 2 tablespoons olive oil
- 1 clove garlic minced
- ½ teaspoon dried basil
- ½ cup shredded parmesan cheese

Directions:

1. Place olive oil in skillet; heat to medium. Add garlic and sauté for one minute.
2. Add green beans to skillet and toss to coat with olive oil.
3. Heat green beans thoroughly and reduce heat to low and cover. Cook beans 5 minutes or until desired tenderness.
4. Place ½ beans on each plate with sliced chicken.
5. Divide parmesan cheese and place ½ on each serving of green beans.

Week 3 Phase 2 **Push** **Monday** Breakfast

Shitake Mushroom and Cheese Omelet with Avocado

Serves Two

Ingredients:

- 4 eggs
- ½ cup shitake mushrooms coarsely chopped
- 2 green onions with stems thinly sliced
- 1 tablespoon chopped parsley
- 2 tablespoons butter (divided for second omelet)
- 3 1 ounce shredded cheddar or crumbled goat cheese (use half for each omelet)
- 1 avocado halved, pitted and peeled
- 2 tablespoons sour cream

Directions:

1. Add eggs to medium bowl and whisk well. Add green onions, and chopped parsley.
2. Heat a skillet to medium high and melt 1 tablespoon butter. Sauté shitake mushrooms along with sliced green onion for 3 or 4 minutes.
3. Remove mushrooms and onions from skillet and place in small bowl. (Skillet with Sloping sides works best for cooking omelets.)
4. Wipe skillet with paper towel and return to medium heat and add 1 tablespoon butter.
5. When the pan is ready, whisk egg mixture one more time before dividing into two equal amounts. Add ½ of the mixture to the skillet. (You may cook the entire mixture into one large omelet, but bear in mind that it is more difficult to handle.)
6. Cook the egg mixture until one side is nearly cooked through, then flip over and spread ½ shredded cheese over omelet. Fold omelet in half and cook for about 30 seconds on one side, then flip omelet over and cook 30 seconds more.
7. Add salt to taste.
8. Place cooked omelet on large plate and prepare second omelet.
9. Slice avocado and place half on each plate and add one tablespoon sour cream on top of each omelet.

Week 3 Phase 2 **Push** **Monday** Lunch

Chicken Flaxseed Wrap with Avocado

Serves Two

Ingredients:

- 2 eggs
- 6 tablespoon ground flaxseeds
- ½ teaspoon baking powder
- ¼ cup grated mozzarella cheese
- 1 tablespoon coconut oil
- 3 tablespoons water
- Pinch of Himalayan pink salt
- 1 tablespoon butter
- 1 cup leftover chicken from Sunday
- 2 tablespoons Hellman's mayonnaise
- 1 cup chopped lettuce
- 1 avocado halved, seeded and peeled
- ¼ medium sliced tomato

Directions:

1. Wisk eggs in a medium-size bowl until well blended. Add ground flaxseed, baking powder, cheese, coconut oil, water and salt and whisk or beat together, blending well.
2. Heat skillet and melt part of butter to grease bottom of skillet.
3. Pour just enough batter to cover the bottom of skillet, keeping it thin like a crepe, being careful not to burn the wrap.
4. You may have to use a spatula to spread out the mixture.
5. Cook for about two minutes and using a spatula, lift wrap onto plate to cool. Make the next wrap.
6. You may make four small wraps or two large wraps.
7. Once wraps are prepared, spread with mayonnaise and divide chicken, avocado, lettuce, and tomato evenly for each wrap.
8. Fold one end up to hold the filling and then fold each side of wrap.

This recipe is so delicious you will want to have it often! I love it!

– Barbara

Week 3 Phase 2 **Push** **Monday** Dinner

Keto Spaghetti and Marinara Meatballs

Serves Four

Keto Spaghetti

Ingredients:

- 1 large spaghetti squash

Directions:

1. Heat oven to 400 degrees.
2. Fill shallow baking dish with two inches of water. Place whole spaghetti squash in the baking dish and place in the middle of the oven.
3. Bake the squash for one hour and check doneness by piercing with a fork.
4. When squash is done remove from the oven and allow cooling before cutting squash in half lengthwise. Scoop out seeds and discard.
5. Using a dinner fork, shred squash into long noodles. Place desired amount of noodles on each plate. Once the meatballs and sauce are ready, place desired amount on top of noodles on each plate.

Marinara and Meatballs

Ingredients

- ¾ pound ground beef
- ¼ pound ground pork (if you don't eat pork add ¼ pound extra beef)
- 1 egg
- ¼ cup grated parmesan cheese
- 2 tablespoons chopped fresh parsley
- ¼ cup chopped onion
- ½ cup shredded mozzarella cheese
- ¼ cup heavy whipping cream
- 1 garlic clove, minced
- ½ teaspoon Himalayan pink salt
- ½ teaspoon pepper
- 2 tablespoons butter or olive oil
- ¼ cup almond flour
- 2 cups low carb or marinara sauce (Rao's is a great low carb product to try and is available at most supermarkets.)

Directions:

1. Add beef, pork, and egg to medium bowl and mix meat and egg together.
2. Add balance of ingredients (except butter and almond flour) to meat and mix to combine, being careful not to over-mix.

Week 3 Phase 2 **Push** **Monday** Dinner... cont

Keto Spaghetti and Marinara Meatballs... cont.

3. Use your hands and shape meat mixture into 10 or 12 small meatballs. *The meatballs do not have a tight consistency as regular meatballs, but be patient as this dish is delicious!*
4. Place the almond flour on a large plate and roll the meatballs in the flour for a light dusting. (Don't be tempted to use more as there are 7 grams of carbs in ¼ cup of almond flour.)
5. Heat a large skillet to medium and melt the butter being careful not to burn. You may use olive oil if you choose.
6. Place meatballs in the skillet and brown. Cook for about 10 minutes.
7. Pour sauce over meatballs and turn heat to low. Allow the meatballs and sauce to merge flavors.
8. Serve over zucchini spaghetti and sprinkle with the desired amount of parmesan cheese. *Yum!*

**Save leftovers for Tuesday lunch.*

NOTES:

Date:

Thoughts: Completing Week 2 and beginning Week 3 Phase 2 Push.

How I'm feeling:

Weight:

Week 3 Phase 2 **Push** **Tuesday** Breakfast

Breakfast Hot Pockets

Serves Two

Ingredients:

- 3 eggs
- 4 slices bacon
- 1/3 cup almond flour
- ¾ cup shredded mozzarella
- 2 tablespoons unsalted butter

Directions:

1. Heat oven to 400 degrees.
2. Place bacon in a large skillet and brown until crisp. Set bacon aside on a paper towel and break into medium size pieces. Drain oil from skillet. Wipe skillet with a paper towel, return to heat and add butter.
3. Whisk eggs in a small bowl and pour into skillet and scramble. Rinse bowl and wipe dry. Place cooked eggs in the bowl and set aside with the bacon.
4. To prepare the dough, melt the shredded mozzarella in the microwave, about 20 or 30 seconds, being careful not to cook the cheese. Combine the almond flour with the melted cheese and mix well to form a dough.
5. Roll the dough between two pieces of wax paper. Your goal is to create two rectangular shaped hot pockets. Grease an oblong cookie sheet with remaining butter. Peel wax paper off the top of wrap and flip it over onto the cookie sheet leaving room for the second wrap. Gently peel off the second piece of wax paper and fill hot pockets with equal parts bacon on each wrap and top with equal parts egg. You may add more shredded mozzarella to your hot pocket if you wish. Fold your hot pocket around filling and place in oven and bake for 20 minutes.
6. Add any seasonings to taste. Hot pockets are great for a variety of fillings.

NOTE: When working with eggs and cheese, it is easy to burn the hot pockets, but they are absolutely delicious and well worth the effort.

Week 3 Phase 2 **Push** **Tuesday** Lunch

Leftover Keto Spaghetti and Marinara Meatballs

Serves Two

From recipe on Page 170 / Monday dinner.

Week 3 Phase 2 **Push** **Tuesday** Dinner

Sautéed Garlic Shrimp with Green Salad and Avocado

Serves Two

Ingredients:

- 1 pound medium size thawed shrimp, tails on or off
- 2 tablespoons olive oil
- 1 tablespoon lemon juice
- 1 large garlic clove crushed
- ¼ teaspoon Himalayan pink salt
- ¼ teaspoon ground black pepper
- 2 tablespoons butter
- 2 tablespoons chopped fresh parsley

Directions:

1. In a large bowl combine all the above ingredients except butter and chopped parsley. Stir and coat ingredients well.
2. In a large skillet add 2 tablespoons butter and melt. Add all coated ingredients and sauté until shrimp is opaque, about 3 to 4 minutes.
3. Serve shrimp over green salad and ½ sliced avocado.
4. You may add two tablespoons of dressing if you choose.

Salad:

1. 1 cup bagged lettuce
2. ½ cup mixed vegetables of your choice
3. 2 tablespoons Ken's low carb ranch or blue cheese dressing

(This dressing is very thick, and you may wish to add one tablespoon olive oil to 2 tablespoons of Ken's.)

Week 3 Phase 2 **Push** **Wednesday** Breakfast

Cheese Scrambled Eggs with Herbs and Bacon

Serves One

Ingredients:

- 2 strips bacon
- 1 tablespoon butter
- 2 eggs
- 2 ounces shredded mozzarella cheese
- 1 tablespoon heavy cream
- ½ teaspoon dried basil
- ½ teaspoon dried thyme
- Salt and pepper to taste

Directions:

1. Add bacon to skillet and cook to desires doneness. Place bacon on plate and remove skillet from heat.
2. In a medium bowl, whisk the eggs with cream and herbs.
3. Melt butter in a medium skillet over low heat and pour egg mixture into the skillet. Top eggs with shredded cheese and stir lightly to keep eggs from browning. Cook eggs to desired doneness and add to plate with bacon.

"By simply deciding exactly what you want, you will begin to move unerringly toward your goal, and your goal will start to move unerringly towards you. At exactly the right place, you and your goal will meet."

— Jack Canfield

Week 3 Phase 2 **Push** **Wednesday** Lunch

Chicken Salad with Magic Puff Bread

Serves Two

Ingredients:

- 2 chicken breasts
- 1 celery rib
- 1 green onion with green top, chopped
- ¼ cup mayo
- 1 teaspoon brown mustard
- 1 teaspoon dill
- 8 pecans or walnuts, broken into small pieces

Directions:

1. Preheat oven to 350 degrees.
2. Coat chicken with olive oil, place in baking dish and put in hot oven.
3. Cook chicken for approximately 30 minutes, depending on thickness of breasts.
4. Watch chicken so it does not dry out or overcook.
5. Remove chicken from oven, cool, and cut into bite sized pieces.
6. In a mixing bowl, except the nuts, combine chicken,
7. celery, mayo, brown mustard, and Himalayan Pink Salt to taste.
8. Using a large spoon, stir all ingredients together until well mixed. Cover and place in frdige to cool and help flavors blend together.
9. Remove Chicken Salad when ready to serve and add chopped nuts, divide between two plates and sprinkle with paprika.

Note: Enjoy with Magic Puff Bread

Magic Puff Bread

Ingredients:

3 eggs

3 tablespoons cream cheese or mascapone, softened

¼ teaspoon cream of tartar

¼ teaspoon salt

Directions:

1. Preheat oven to 300 degrees.
2. Using two bowls, separate egg whites from yolks. Add cream of tartar and salt to the bowl of egg whites. Mix egg whites using a hand-held mixer until stiff peaks form.
3. In bowl of egg yolks, add softened cream cheese or mascarpone cheese and mix together until well-blended.
4. Take the yolk mixture and pour slowly into egg whites using a rubber spatula to gently fold ingredients together.

Week 3 Phase 2 **Push** **Wednesday** Lunch... cont.

Chicken Salad with Magic Puff Bread... cont. **Serves Four**

5. Place parchment paper on large baking pan with sides so batter doesn't flow over the sides into oven. Using a medium sized ladle, pour mixture onto parchment paper creating 6 circular disc.
6. Place on middle rack in oven and bake for 30 minutes until disc are golden brown.
7. Allow them to cool so they do not fall apart.

Magic Puff Bread makes amazing sandwiches and the carb count is a whopping 0.2! So, don't hesitate to use two pieces. Store bread in a zip lock bag and put in fridge.

– Barbara

Week 3 Phase 2 **Push** **Wednesday** Dinner

Keto Sausage Pizza

Serves Two

Pizza Dough Ingredients:

- Preheat oven to 400 degrees
- 2 cups shredded mozzarella cheese
- 1 tablespoon psyllium husk powder
- ¾ cup almond flour
- 3 tablespoons cream cheese
- 1 egg
- 1 tablespoon Italian seasoning
- 1 tablespoon olive oil

Pizza Topping Ingredients:

- ½ cup Rao's marinara
- 1 cup shredded mozzarella cheese
- ½ teaspoon oregano
- 1 small can sliced mushrooms
- ¼ pound cooked crumbled sausage (You may substitute pepperoni or ham)

Directions:

1. Place mozzarella cheese in medium microwave dish and melt cheese, about 20 to 30 seconds. Be careful not to cook the mozzarella. Add all the other pizza dough ingredients except the olive oil. Work mixture into a ball with hands or a fork.
2. Place olive oil on your hands and completely coat pizza dough. Spread dough evenly on pizza pan.
3. Place pizza crust in 400-degree oven and bake for 10 minutes. Remove crust from oven and carefully flip over, using a large flat spatula to keep from separating crust. Place back in the oven for additional 3 minutes.
4. Remove crust from oven and add Rao's low carb marinara sauce, spreading evenly over pizza.
5. Spread mozzarella cheese over sauce and sprinkle oregano over pizza. Spread mushrooms and crumbled sausage evenly over pizza.
6. Place pizza in the oven for additional 4 or 5 minutes. Remove from oven, cool and serve.

Week 3 Phase 2 **Push** **Thursday** Breakfast

Coconut Chia Oatmeal

Serves Four

Ingredients:

**Prepare this dish the night before.*

- 1 ¾ cup water
- 1 cup unsweetened coconut milk
- 1 teaspoon vanilla
- ½ cup chia seeds
- ¼ cup unsweetened shredded coconut
- ¼ cup walnut pieces or slivered almonds
- 2 drops liquid stevia
- ¼ cup blueberries
- 1 small carton heavy whipping cream

Directions:

1. Pour water and coconut milk in a medium bowl and stir in chia seeds, coconut, nuts, and vanilla. Stir ingredients well to blend.
2. Cover the Coconut Chia Oatmeal and place in the fridge overnight to allow the chia seeds to soak up the liquid.
3. In the morning remove the oatmeal from the refrigerator and divide into four bowls. Add fruit and whip cream.
4. Place whipping cream and 2 drops of stevia in a medium bowl and beat until fluffy.

**I like to heat the berries for 20 seconds in the microwave to make them warm and juicy! You may add 2 drops of stevia to sweeten berries if you wish.*

"Change is the constant, the signal for rebirth, the egg of the phoenix."
— Christina Baldwin

Week 3 Phase 2 **Push** **Thursday** Lunch

Crabmeat Stuffed Avocado with Green Salad

Serves Two

Ingredients:

- 2 tablespoons mayonnaise
- 1 four ounces can lump crab-meat
- 1 teaspoon lime juice
- ½ teaspoon cumin
- Dash of paprika
- ¼ cup chopped celery
- 1 medium avocado
- 1 cup salad greens of your choice

Directions:

1. Open and drain liquid from crabmeat. In a medium bowl combine crabmeat, mayonnaise, lime juice, cumin, paprika, and celery. Mix well.
2. Slice avocado in two lengthwise, pit, and peel.
3. Add salad greens to two plates and place one-half avocados on each plate. Divide crab mixture in two and place a rounded scoop in each half avocado.

This recipe is so delicious you will want to have it often! I love it!

– Barbara

Week 3 Phase 2 **Push** **Thursday** Dinner

Pork Loin Roast with Cheesy Mock Mashed Potato and Salad

Serves Two

Ingredients:

- Preheat oven to 350 degrees
- ¼ cup balsamic vinegar
- 2 tablespoons Montreal Steak Seasoning
- 3 tablespoon olive oil
- 1 garlic clove, minced
- 2 pounds boneless pork loin
- ½ teaspoon Himalayan pink salt
- Ground black pepper to taste

Directions:

1. Stir together balsamic vinegar, Montreal Steak Seasoning, olive oil, and minced garlic.
2. Place pork roast in shallow roasting pan and spread olive oil and herb mixture over roast. Place roast in preheated oven for 1 hour. Roast should be done when an oven thermometer reaches 145 degrees.

Cheesy Mock Mashed Potato

See Ingredients and Directions on Page 138.

Salad:

1. 1 cup bagged lettuce
2. ½ cup mixed vegetables of your choice
3. 2 tablespoons Ken's low carb ranch or blue cheese dressing

(This dressing is very thick, and you may wish to add one tablespoon olive oil to 2 tablespoons of Ken's.)

Week 3 Phase 2 **Push** **Friday** Breakfast

Coconut Almond Pancakes

Serves Two

Ingredients:

- 3 tablespoon butter
- ½ cup heavy whipping cream
- ¼ teaspoon vanilla
- 2 drops liquid stevia
- 4 large eggs
- ⅓ cup Philadelphia brand cream cheese
- ¼ cup coconut flour
- ¼ cup almond flour
- ¼ teaspoon nutmeg
- 1 teaspoon cinnamon
- 2 drops liquid stevia
- ⅓ to ½ cup full-fat coconut milk
- ½ teaspoon vanilla
- ⅓ cup walnut pieces, (optional)
- ¼ cup blueberries

Directions:

- In a medium bowl, add the whipping cream and 2 drops of stevia and ¼ teaspoon vanilla. Whip until fluffy. Place in fridge until pancakes are ready.
- Heat pancake griddle to medium. You may use a large skillet if you choose.
- In another medium bowl, add 4 eggs and cream cheese and beat with small handheld mixer. Add flour, nutmeg, cinnamon, stevia, and coconut milk to mixture and blend well. If mixture is too thick add more coconut milk to desired consistency. Add vanilla and whisk until well blended.
- Stir in walnut pieces.
- Add half of butter to griddle and melt. Pour desired amount of batter to hot griddle and cook until top starts to bubble. Flip pancakes over and continue cooking until done. Watch carefully not to burn the butter.
- Heat blueberries and 2 drops stevia in microwave for 15 seconds. It makes them warm and juicy.
- Place pancakes on plates and add butter, blueberries and whipped cream.

Week 3 Phase 2 **Push** **Friday** Lunch

Cream of Broccoli and Spinach Soup

Serves Two

Ingredients:

- 2 tablespoons butter
- 1 small carton pre-chopped onion
- 1 small carton pre-chopped celery
- 2 cloves garlic, crushed
- 1 head broccoli chopped
- 3 cups regular organic chicken stock
- 1 small bag fresh baby spinach
- ¼ cup sour cream
- ½ cup fresh basil, chopped
- ¼ teaspoon Ground Cayenne Red Pepper
- Himalayan pink salt to taste
- Ground black pepper to taste

Directions:

1. In a large soup pot, melt butter and sauté onion, celery, and garlic.
2. Chop broccoli into small florets and chop the upper part of the stalk and add to pot.
3. Pour in chicken stock and bring to a boil. (Do not use low-fat.)
4. Add spinach to boiling stock.
5. Continue boiling ingredients for 15 minutes.
6. Remove from heat and add sour cream and basil.
7. Add red pepper (optional).
8. Taste soup and add salt and pepper as needed.
9. Ladle soup to bowls and add a dollop of sour cream to each if you like.
10. Feel free to spice it up any way you choose.

Week 3 Phase 2 **Push** **Friday** Dinner

Steak and Asparagus Salad

Serves Two

Ingredients:

- 1 pound tenderloin or sirloin steak
- ¼ teaspoon Montreal steak seasoning
- ¼ teaspoon Himalayan pink salt
- ½ teaspoon ground black pepper
- 1 garlic clove, minced
- 1 pound asparagus trimmed
- 2 tablespoons chopped fresh basil
- 1 tablespoon lemon juice
- 2 tablespoons olive oil
- 1 teaspoon capers, drained and rinsed

Directions:

1. Season steak with Montreal steak seasoning, salt, pepper, and garlic.
2. Broil or grill steak to desired doneness.
3. Steam or sauté asparagus until tender. Drain and chop asparagus into two-inch pieces. In a large bowl combine asparagus, basil, and lemon juice. Mix well and divide between two plates.
4. In a small bowl add olive oil and capers. Mash capers into olive oil. You may use a small food processor if you wish.
5. Slice steak into strips and divide between two plates. Place steak on top of asparagus and drizzle olive oil and capers over steaks.

This is one of my favorite dishes!
– Barbara

Week 3 Phase 2 **Push** **Saturday** Breakfast

Poached Eggs, Sautéed Spinach and Canadian Bacon with Hollandaise Sauce

Serves Two

Ingredients:

- 4 eggs
- 4 slices Canadian bacon
- 1 tablespoon olive oil
- 1 tablespoon butter
- 1 bag prewashed spinach
- 1 garlic clove crushed
- Himalayan pink salt and pepper to taste

Directions:

1. Add water to egg poaching pan and heat to boiling. Oil egg cups with olive oil and place eggs in egg cups and cover pan. It could take 8 to 10 minutes to cook the eggs.
2. Wait 5 minutes for the eggs to start cooking before heating the skillet. Add olive oil to skillet and heat to medium. Add Canadian bacon and lightly brown. Remove from pan and place two slices per plate.
3. Wipe skillet clean and melt butter. Add crushed garlic to butter and sauté. Add spinach to skillet and stir until wilted. Place cooked spinach on top of bacon.
4. Remove eggs from egg poacher and scoop on top of spinach.
5. Add salt and pepper.

Keto Hollandaise Sauce

Ingredients:

- 3 egg yolks
- ½ cup butter
- 1 tablespoon lemon juice
- Himalayan pink salt and pepper to taste
- Dash of cayenne (optional)

Directions:

1. Place egg yolks in food processor or blender.
2. Melt the butter in microwave until bubbling, being careful not to brown.
3. With the food processor running, gradually pour hot butter into egg yolks. This will create a thick sauce. Add lemon juice, salt, pepper, and cayenne. Pour hollandaise over poached eggs.

Week 3 Phase 2 **Push** **Saturday** Lunch

Roasted Brussels Sprouts

Serves Two

Ingredients:

- 1 pound medium-sized Brussels sprouts
- 4 slices crispy bacon
- ¼ cup butter or olive oil
- ¼ cup grated parmesan cheese
- ½ teaspoon Himalayan pink salt
- Ground black pepper to taste

**Feel free to add any seasonings you wish.*

Directions:

1. Preheat oven to 375 degrees.
2. Brown bacon slices, cool and break into small pieces.
3. Wash and cut Brussels sprouts in half, melt butter and pour over Brussels sprouts. Add bacon pieces evenly over sprouts.
4. Sprinkle with parmesan cheese, salt, and pepper.
5. Place on baking sheet and roast for approximately 30 minutes. Check baking progress to avoid over browning sprouts.
6. You may add a small salad if you wish.

Salad:

1. 1 cup bagged lettuce
2. ½ cup mixed vegetables of your choice
3. 2 tablespoons Ken's low carb ranch or blue cheese dressing

(This dressing is very thick, and you may wish to add one tablespoon olive oil to 2 tablespoons of Ken's.)

Week 3 Phase 2 **Push** **Saturday** Dinner

Pan-Fried Trout with Baked Sweet Potato and Salad

Serves Two

Ingredients:

- 2 medium sweet potatoes
- 2 trout fillets with skin on
- 4 tablespoons butter
- 2 garlic cloves, crushed
- 4 tablespoons chopped fresh parsley
- 1 tablespoon lemon juice
- Himalayan pink salt to taste
- Ground black pepper to taste

Directions:

1. Preheat oven to 400 degrees.
2. Wash and dry sweet potatoes, wrap with foil and place in hot oven. Bake for approximately 45 minutes to 1 hour depending on the size of sweet potatoes.
3. When sweet potatoes are done, remove from oven and leave wrapped in foil until fish is ready.
4. Heat a large non-stick skillet to medium and melt butter until bubbly. Add trout skin side down, add garlic, fresh parsley, lemon juice, salt and pepper, and cook for 5 or 6 minutes or until fish is cooked through. Cook time will depend on the thickness of trout fillets.
5. Place fish on large dinner plates and unwrap sweet potato and place on plate with fish. Slice sweet potato open lengthwise and add a tablespoon of butter to each.

Salad:

1. 1 cup bagged lettuce
2. ½ cup mixed vegetables of your choice
3. 2 tablespoons Ken's low carb ranch or blue cheese dressing

(This dressing is very thick, and you may wish to add one tablespoon olive oil to 2 tablespoons of Ken's.)

Week 3 Phase 2 **Push** **Sunday** Breakfast

English Style Breakfast

Serves One

Ingredients:

- Two large eggs
- Two tablespoons butter or olive oil
- Two slices ham
- One link sausage
- One half cup mushrooms
- One plum tomato
- One half sliced avocado
- Salt and pepper to taste

Directions:

1. Melt butter in large skillet on low heat.
2. Add ham, sausage, mushrooms to skillet and sauté.
3. Slice tomato lengthwise and place in skillet cut side down in butter.
4. Push everything to side with spatula and add eggs.
5. Cook eggs to desired doneness and place on plate.
6. Add ham, mushrooms, sausage, and tomato.
7. Add sliced avocado to plate.
8. Add salt and pepper to taste.

"Don't let the noise of others opinions drown out your own inner voice, and most important, have the courage to follow your heart and intuition. They somehow already know what you truly want to become."

— Steve Jobs

Week 3 Phase 2 **Push** **Sunday** Lunch

Greek Salad

Serves Two

Ingredients:

- ½ medium cucumber cut lengthwise and sliced
- 1 tomato sliced in small wedges
- ½ medium red pepper, sliced
- 4 green onions, sliced using part of stem
- 12 Kalamata olives, pitted
- 1 teaspoon oregano
- ⅓ cup olive oil
- 1 tablespoon balsamic vinegar
- 2 thick slices fresh feta cheese

Directions:

1. Divide all ingredients into two equal amounts except olive oil, balsamic, and feta cheese.
2. Add balsamic to olive oil and pore over above ingredients.
3. Place on two salad plates.
4. Add one feta cheese slice to each plate.
5. Add salt and pepper to taste.
6. Enjoy with Lamb Burgers or go meatless.

This recipe is so delicious you will want to have it often! I love it!

– Barbara

Week 3 Phase 2 **Push** **Sunday** Dinner

Chicken Breasts Stuffed with Artichoke Hearts and Goat Cheese with Garlic Green Beans

Serves Four

Ingredients:

- 3 tablespoons olive oil
- 1 cup canned chopped artichoke hearts in water
- ¼ cup shallots, minced
- ¼ cup crumbled goat cheese
- 1 teaspoon herbs de Provence (you may substitute thyme)
- ¼ teaspoon Himalayan pink salt
- ¼ teaspoon ground black pepper
- Four boned chicken breast halves
- 1 cup low sodium chicken broth
- Two tablespoons lemon juice
- Two teaspoons almond flour
- Chopped fresh parsley for garnish

Directions:

1. Add one tablespoon olive oil to large non-stick skillet and heat to medium. Add chopped artichokes and minced shallot to skillet and sauté for 4 minutes. Remove artichokes and shallots from pan and place in a bowl to cool. Stir in goat cheese and half of Herbs de Provence, salt, and pepper. Set aside.
2. Rinse and dry chicken breasts. Cut a slice in chicken breasts to create a pocket. Divide artichoke mixture into equal parts for each breast. Stuff mixture into each pocket.
3. Return non-stick skillet to medium heat and add 1 tablespoon olive oil. Place chicken in skillet and sprinkle with remaining salt and pepper. Cook chicken breasts for 6 minutes on each side, carefully turning over. Cut into the chicken to assure it is cooked through. Remove chicken breasts from pan and place on large platter and set aside.
4. Add balance of Herbs de Provence to skillet and add chicken broth, and bring to a boil. Reduce to medium.
5. Stir in lemon juice and almond flour and blend well. Cook until broth thickens. Add chicken to skillet, cover and cook 5 minutes until thoroughly heated and flavors are well-blended.
6. Place chicken breasts on plates and top with equal amounts sauce. Garnish with fresh parsley.

Week 3 Phase 2 **Push** **Sunday** Dinner

Chicken Breasts Stuffed with Artichoke Hearts and Goat Cheese with Garlic Green Beans...cont.

Serves Four

Parmesan Garlic Green Beans

Ingredients:

- One pound fresh green beans, trimmed
- Two tablespoons olive oil
- Two garlic cloves, minced
- Four tablespoons chopped walnuts
- ¼ cup grated parmesan cheese

Directions:

1. Bring a large pot of water to a boil and carefully place green beans in pot. Cover pot and cook greens beans for 5 minutes or until tender.
2. Drain green beans in colander and set aside.
3. In a large skillet, heat the olive oil. Place garlic and walnuts in hot skillet and sauté.
4. Add green beans to skillet, sprinkle with parmesan cheese, and sauté.

NOTES

This is the end of Week 3. My self assessment of the past three weeks:

List the positive actions I completed to help myself get this far:

Week 4 Final Phase 2 **Finish Line** **Monday** Breakfast

Sautéed Vegetables with Scrambled Eggs

Serves One

Ingredients

- 2 tablespoons olive oil
- 2 large eggs
- ¼ red pepper, chopped
- ¼ onion, chopped
- 1 cup fresh spinach leaves
- Salt and pepper to taste

Directions:

1. Add olive oil to skillet and heat low to medium.
2. Scramble eggs in small bowl and set aside.
3. Add red pepper and onion to skillet and sauté.
4. Once vegetables are soft, add in spinach.
5. Stir in spinach
6. Add scrambled eggs and stir until cooked.

NOTES

Date:

Starting Week 4 Final Phase Finish Line — What are my thoughts?

Wow! I've gotten this far. How do I feel?

Weight:

Week 4 Final Phase 2 **Finish Line** **Monday** Lunch

Kale Sausage Pattie with Salad

Serves Two

Ingredients:

- ½ 2 tablespoons olive oil
- ½ cup chopped or finely shredded kale
- ½ cup chopped fresh mushrooms
- 1 clove garlic, crushed
- ½ pound ground pork
- ¼ cup shredded mozzarella cheese
- ½ teaspoon Himalayan Pink Salt

Directions:

1. Melt one tablespoon olive oil in large skillet.
2. Place kale, mushroom and garlic in skillet and sauté until cooked.
3. Remove from heat and place vegetables in a mixing bowl.
4. Add the ground pork and cheese to vegetables and mix well.
5. Form pork and vegetable mix into four sausage patties.
6. Add one tablespoon olive oil to skillet and add sausage patties. Cook on low to keep patties from over browning

Salad

Ingredients:

- ½ sliced tomato
- 1 avocado, peeled and seeded
- Salt and pepper to taste
- Sliced green onion
- 2 tablespoons olive oil
- 1 teaspoon balsamic vinegar
- ½ Salt and pepper to taste

Directions:

1. Divide tomato, avocado and onion on two small salad plates.
2. Mix olive oil and vinegar and pour over salads.
3. Add salt and pepper to taste.

Week 4 Final Phase 2 **Finish Line** **Monday** Dinner

Parmesan Crusted Chicken and Baked Sweet Potato

Serves Two

Ingredients:

- Pre-heat oven to 425 degrees
- 4 chicken breast halves
- ½ cup Hellmann's Real Mayonnaise
- ¼ cup grated parmesan cheese
- ½ tsp. Italian Seasoning
- ½ cup finely crushed pork rind

Directions:

1. Line baking sheet with foil for easy cleanup. Place chicken on baking sheet.
2. Mix mayonnaise, parmesan cheese, and Italian seasoning together.
3. Spread mixture evenly over chicken and coat with pork rind by pressing it into mayonnaise and cheese mixture.
4. Place chicken in oven and bake for 20 to 25 minutes depending on thickness of chicken.

Baked Sweet Potato

Ingredients:

- 2 small sweet potatoes or one large one shared
- 2 tablespoons full fat butter for each potato.
- You may bake or microwave potatoes.

Note: You can now purchase small sweet potatoes in a microwave wrapper that works great and only takes 6 to 8 minutes.

Directions:

To bake the sweet potato:

1. Heat oven to 400 degrees.
2. Wrap sweet potato in foil and secure tightly.
3. Place on middle rack and bake for 40 minutes for medium potato, or for 1 hour for large potato.

It's a wonderful dish!

– Barbara

Week 4 Final Phase 2 **Finish Line** **Tuesday** Breakfast

Tomato Omelet with Goat Cheese

Serves One

Ingredients:

- 2 large eggs
- 1 tablespoon cream or full fat milk
- ¼ chopped tomato
- ½ ounce crumbled goat cheese
- 1 tablespoon butter or olive oil
- 1 green onion, chopped

Directions:

1. Heat medium non-stick skillet on low heat and add butter.
2. Whisk eggs and cream together in small bowl.
3. Add egg mixture to heated skillet and let spread out by tilting pan slightly. Cook until egg mixture is solid, about 1 or 2 minutes.
4. Add goat cheese and tomatoes to eggs and fold over to create an omelet. You may flip the omelet over to cook on other side if you wish.
5. Garnish with chopped green onion. (Note) You may add a tablespoon of sour cream or salsa if you wish.

"I am learning that if I just go on accepting the framework for life that others have given me, if I fail to make my own choices, the reason for my life will be missing. I will be unable to recognize that which I have the power to change."
— Liv Ullmann

Week 4 Final Phase 2 **Finish Line** **Tuesday** Lunch

Cheeseburger Salad

Serves Two

Ingredients:

- 4 tablespoons olive or avocado oil
- ½ pound ground beef
- ½ teaspoon garlic salt
- ¼ teaspoon black pepper
- ½ teaspoon Himalayan Pink Salt
- Dash of red pepper flakes, optional
- 2 thick slices white onion
- 2 medium slices tomato

Directions:

1. In a large bowl combine ground beef, garlic salt, pepper, pink salt, pepper flakes. Mix together well to combine ingredients. Shape beef mixture into two patties.
2. Place the olive oil in a large skillet and heat on medium high.
3. Reduce heat to medium and add patties to hot oil in skillet, being careful oil it not too hot. Cook 2 or 3 minutes on each side or until desired doneness. Reduce heat to low if patties are over-browning.
4. Add a slice of cheddar or American cheese if desired.
5. Place one cheeseburger on each plate and add a slice of tomato and slice of onion on top.
6. Add condiments, but be careful with ketchup as it is loaded with sugar! Mustard and Hellman's Mayonnaise are good choices.

Week 4 Final Phase 2 **Finish Line** **Tuesday** Dinner

Keto Shrimp Scampi and Spaghetti Squash with Salad

Serves Two

Ingredients:

- 1 medium spaghetti squash
- 3 tablespoons olive oil
- 3 tablespoons butter
- 1-pound uncooked shrimp (peeled, deveined, and tails removed.
- ¼ cup grated parmesan cheese
- 2 garlic cloves, crushed
- Pinch red pepper flakes
- ½ teaspoon Himalayan Pink Salt
- ½ teaspoon black pepper
- ½ cup dry white wine
- 2 tablespoons chopped fresh parsley

Directions:

1. Prepare spaghetti squash by puncturing holes in several places and then placing it in the microwave. Microwave for approximately 10 to 12 minutes.
2. Remove squash when done and carefully slice off the ends to release steam. Let sit while you prepare shrimp dish.
3. Place olive oil in a large skillet and heat to medium high.
4. Add all the ingredients except wine and spaghetti squash.
5. Cook approximately 10 minutes or until shrimp are cooked through.
6. Stir in wine and remove pan from heat and let sit.
7. Slice spaghetti squash lengthwise and remove seeds, scoop out center and discard. Shred squash with fork to form noodles. Divide noodles on two places.
8. Spoon shrimp mixture onto spaghetti noodles and enjoy.
9. Note: If you choose to use frozen pre-cooked shrimp, the shrimp will be tough and not as flavorful.

Salad:

- 1 cup bagged lettuce
- ½ cup mixed vegetables of your choice
- 2 tablespoons Ken's low carb ranch or blue cheese dressing

(This dressing is very thick, and you may wish to add one tablespoon olive oil to 2 tablespoons of Ken's.)

Week 4 Final Phase 2 **Finish Line** **Wednesday** Breakfast

Keto Almond and Cream Cheese Pancakes

Serves Two

Ingredients:

- 2/3 cup almond flour
- ½ cup softened Philadelphia original cream cheese
- 2 large eggs
- ½ teaspoon cinnamon
- 1 tablespoon butter for frying
- ½ cup whipping cream (If you have lactose issues you may use a sugar free syrup, such as, Lakanto Maple Flavored Syrup.)
- 2 drops stevia
- 1 teaspoon vanilla

Directions:

1. Pour whipping cream in medium size bowl and using handheld mixer, whip until thick and fluffy. Add 2 drops of Stevia and one teaspoon vanilla and blend. Set aside.
2. Combine almond flour, cream cheese, eggs and cinnamon in medium size bowl and mix with hand held mixer until well blended.
3. Add butter to non-stick frying pan and heat to medium.
4. Pour in a quarter cup batter to heated pan and cook until pancake starts to bubble. Flip pancake over to cook on other side. Continue cooking pancakes.
5. Top pancakes with whipped cream or Lakanto Maple Flavored Syrup. This is a sugar free Keto friendly syrup and has over 1500 reviews on Amazon. I ordered mine on Amazon.

Week 4 Final Phase 2 **Finish Line** **Wednesday** Lunch

Wedge Salad with Grilled Chicken

Serves Two

Preheat Oven to 350 degrees

Blue Cheese Dressing

Ingredients:

- ½ cup full fat sour cream
- ¼ cup mayonnaise
- 2 tablespoons buttermilk
- 2 teaspoons red wine vinegar
- ¼ teaspoon Worcestershire sauce
- ½ teaspoon garlic salt
- Salt and pepper to taste
- 2 ounces blue cheese

Directions:

1. Simply add all the above ingredients together in a small bowl, stir well to create the desired consistency. You may add extra buttermilk to create a creamier dressing. Place in fridge to cool while preparing salad.

Salad

Ingredients:

- ½ pound baked chicken strips
- 2 tablespoon olive oil
- 1 small head of lettuce
- 4 slices bacon
- ¾ cup cherry tomatoes
- ¼ cup chopped onion
- Salt and pepper to taste

Directions:

1. Place chicken strips on a cookie sheet with sides to prevent dripping into oven. Coat chicken with olive oil, and salt and pepper to taste. Place in oven on middle rack and bake for approximately 20 minutes. If you wish to save time, cut the chicken into small bite size pieces. It is not necessary to flip the chicken.
2. While the chicken is baking, cook 4 slices of bacon in a skillet until crispy. Remove from pan when fully cooked and set aside to cool.
3. Choose two large plates and cut head of lettuce in two and use only one section to cut in half again creating 2 wedges. You may save the other half. Place the two wedges on the plates.
4. Remove the blue cheese dressing from fridge and divide between the two salads. Sprinkle with desired salt and black pepper. Add the cherry tomatoes and onion on top of dressing, adding crumbled bacon and extra blue cheese if you wish.
5. Remove baked chicken from oven, cool slightly and place on the salad.

Week 4 Final Phase 2 **Finish Line** **Wednesday** Dinner

Keto Italian Pizza

Serves Four

Ingredients:

- Preheat oven to 425 degrees
- ¾ cup finely ground almond flour
- 2 cups shredded full-fat mozzarella cheese
- ¼ cup cream cheese
- ½ cup mozzarella cheese for topping

Directions:

1. Place the almond flour and cheese in a large sauce pan and stir mixture over low heat. Remove from heat when mixture starts to form a dough.
2. Roll dough between two pieces of parchment paper approximately 14 inches long.
3. Dough should be rolled into a circle about 12 inches in diameter.
4. Carefully peel off the top piece of parchment and slide the circle onto a pizza pan, leaving the bottom piece under the dough.
5. To keep the dough from shrinking, poke holes using a fork.
6. Place pizza dough on the center rack of oven and bake for approximately 8 minutes, watching carefully not to burn crust.
7. Remove pizza crust from oven and place on cutting board or towel. Reduce heat to 350 degrees.
8. Add Rau's Pizza Sauce and spread evenly over crust.
9. Sprinkle ¼ cup parmesan cheese over pizza sauce.
10. Add your favorite ingredients, but no pineapple, as it is full of sugar. You may add hot pepper corns, jalapenos, mushrooms, pepperoni, ham, onion, green or red pepper, and extra mozzarella cheese.
11. Place back in the oven just long enough to heat toppings.
12. Remove from oven and let slightly cool before slicing pizza.

Note: This pizza dough is not pliable like traditional pizza dough. It is better to slice and slide your pizza wedge onto a plate and eat using a fork.

Week 4 Final Phase 2 **Finish Line** **Thursday** Breakfast

Spicy Fried Eggs and Bacon

Serves Two

Ingredients:

- 4 large eggs
- Pinch ground cumin
- Pinch garlic salt
- Pinch chili powder
- Pinch paprika
- Pinch Himalayan Pink Salt
- 1 tablespoon butter
- 4 strips bacon

Note: Greenfield Natural Meat Company makes the best uncured bacon I have ever had. It boasts no antibiotics or growth hormones,100% vegetarian and gluten free. I highly recommend this bacon. It is delicious.

Directions:

1. Heat large skillet to medium high and add 4 strips of bacon. Fry bacon to desired crispiness and place two pieces on each plate.
2. Combine the spices together in a small bowl.
3. Wipe out frying pan and return to heat.
4. Add butter to pan and bring to medium heat.
5. Add 4 eggs and reduce heat to low to prevent burning or over browning of eggs.
6. When whites are cooked through, gently flip eggs and cook a few seconds or until desired doneness.
7. Carefully lift eggs from pan and place two eggs on each plate.
8. Sprinkle as much spice mix on eggs as desired.

Note: You may add hot sauce to your eggs if you wish.

Week 4 Final Phase 2 **Finish Line** **Thursday** Lunch

Cheesy Ground Beef Soup

Serves Two

Ingredients:

- 4 slices bacon
- 1-pound ground beef
- 1 tablespoon butter
- 1 small carton chopped white onion
- 1 carton chopped celery
- 1 teaspoon basil
- 2 garlic cloves, crushed
- 1 cup cauliflower broken into small florets
- 1 cup broccoli cut into small pieces
- 1 8-ounce bag shredded sharp cheddar cheese
- 3 cups chicken stock
- 1 cup heavy whipping cream
- ¾ cup shredded sharp cheddar cheese
- Himalayan Pink Salt (Note: Be careful on the salt as the cheese has a lot of salt.)
- Ground black pepper to taste
- ¼ cup sour cream

Directions:

1. Heat skillet to medium high. Add the bacon and cook until crispy. Remove the bacon and place on paper towel to cool.
2. Leave the bacon fat in the skillet, add ground beef and brown.
3. Remove from burner, leave ground beef in skillet and set aside.
4. Heat large soup pot to medium. Add 2 tablespoons butter or olive oil.
5. Add onions, and garlic and sauté for 2 or 3 minutes until softened.
6. Add broccoli and cauliflower. Sauté for 3 or 4 minutes, being careful not to burn the bottom.
7. Break bacon into pieces and add along with browned ground beef. Note: Save one strip bacon, crumble and set aside for garnish.
8. Add chicken stock and bring to boil.
9. Reduce heat to low and cook approximately 20 minutes until all ingredients are tender. (Note: Occasionally check to ensure mixture is not burning onto the bottom of the pot.)
10. Add cheese, heavy whipping cream, salt and pepper. Stir cheese constantly to melt and reduce heat to simmer.
11. Stir in the sour cream.
12. Spoon into 2 bowls and top with extra cheddar cheese and crumbled bacon bits.

Note: This soup is absolutely delicious and should be left on simmer for an additional half hour to blend the flavors. It tastes even better the next day!

Week 4 Final Phase 2 **Finish Line** **Thursday** Dinner

Garlic Butter Steak with Shitake Mushrooms

Serves Two

Ingredients:

- 2 boneless sirloin or New York Strip, or steak of your choice any thickness you choose.
- ½ pound fresh shitake mushrooms, thinly sliced
- ½ pound asparagus, trimmed
- 3 tablespoons olive oil
- 2 tablespoons organic butter
- Himalayan Pink Salt
- Freshly ground black pepper
- ½ teaspoon Montreal Steak Seasoning
- 2 cloves garlic, minced
- 1 tablespoon finely chopped fresh rosemary

Directions:

Note: This dish is best prepared in a cast iron skillet.

1. Heat cast iron skillet on high heat until skillet is extremely hot.
2. Add two tablespoons olive oil to hot pan and coat one tablespoon oil on steak. Season steak with salt, pepper, and Montreal Steak Seasoning.
3. Reduce heat to medium and sear for about 5 minutes on one side to seal in juices. Turn steaks over carefully so as not to splatter olive oil. Continue cooking steaks.
4. Add butter to pan and spread it all around the steaks add the garlic. Baste some of the butter on top of the steaks.
5. Spread mushrooms and trimmed asparagus around the steaks and cook for 5 minutes longer. If you want your steak rare, you may remove from the pan any time you wish.
6. Using two large dinner plates, place a steak on each, divide mushrooms and asparagus and add to each plate. Using any drippings from pan, carefully pour over each plate.

Week 4 Final Phase 2 **Finish Line** **Friday** Breakfast

Mushroom and Egg Frittata

Serves Four

Ingredients:

- 8 eggs
- ½ cup heavy whipping cream
- 1 cup canned sliced mushrooms
- 1 green onion finely sliced
- Salt and pepper to taste
- ¼ cup grated Parmesan cheese
- 2 tablespoons butter

Directions:

1. In a large mixing bowl, add eggs and mix on low using a handheld mixer.
2. Add whipping cream and mix together with eggs.
3. Add balance of ingredients to egg mixture and mix together for a few seconds.
4. Heat large skillet to medium high, add butter, and when melted, add egg mixture into hot pan.
5. Reduce heat to low so as not to burn frittata, and continue cooking until eggs are fully cooked.
6. Divide onto 4 large plates and serve.

Note: If you are serving only 2, just refrigerate half of dish for another meal.

"Courage, like fear is a habit. The more you do it, the more you do it, and this habit—of stepping up, of taking action—more than anything else, will move you in a different direction."

— Tony Robbins

Week 4 Final Phase 2 **Finish Line** **Friday** Lunch

Chicken Salad with Magic Puff Bread

Serves Two

Ingredients:

- 2 chicken breasts
- 1 celery rib
- 1 green onion with green top, chopped
- ¼ cup mayo
- 1 teaspoon brown mustard
- 1 teaspoon dill
- 8 pecans or walnuts, broken into small pieces

Directions:

1. Preheat oven to 350 degrees.
2. Coat chicken with olive oil, place in baking dish and put in hot oven.
3. Cook chicken for approximately 30 minutes, depending on thickness of breasts.
4. Watch chicken so it does not dry out or overcook.
5. Remove chicken from oven, cool, and cut into bite sized pieces.
6. In a mixing bowl, except the nuts, combine chicken, celery, mayo, brown mustard, and Himalayan Pink Salt to taste.
7. Using a large spoon, stir all ingredients together until well mixed. Cover and place in fridge to cool and help flavors blend together.
8. Remove Chicken Salad when ready to serve and add chopped nuts, divide between two plates and sprinkle with paprika.

Note: Enjoy with Magic Puff Bread

Magic Puff Bread

Ingredients:

1. 3 eggs
2. 3 tablespoons cream cheese or mascapone, softened
3. ¼ teaspoon cream of tartar
4. ¼ teaspoon salt

Directions:

1. Preheat oven to 300 degrees.
2. Using two bowls, separate egg whites from yolks. Add cream of tartar and salt to the bowl of egg whites. Mix egg whites using a hand-held mixer until stiff peaks form.
3. In bowl of egg yolks, add softened cream cheese or mascarpone cheese and mix together until well-blended.
4. Take the yolk mixture and pour slowly into egg whites using a rubber spatula to gently fold

Week 4 Final Phase 2 **Finish Line** **Friday ... cont.** Lunch ...cont.

Chicken Salad with Magic Puff Bread... cont.

ingredients together.

5. Place parchment paper on large baking pan with sides so batter doesn't flow over the sides into oven. Using a medium sized ladle, pour mixture onto parchment paper creating 6 circular disc.
6. Place on middle rack in oven and bake for 30 minutes until disc are golden brown.
7. Allow them to cool so they do not fall apart.

Magic Puff Bread makes amazing sandwiches and the carb count is a whopping 0.2! So, don't hesitate to use two pieces. Store bread in a zip lock bag and put in fridge.

– Barbara

Week 4 Final Phase 2 **Finish Line** **Friday** Dinner

Keto Pork Chops with Blue Cheese Sauce

Serves Two

Ingredients:

- 2 bone in pork chops
- 2 tablespoons butter or olive oil
- Himalayan Pink Salt and pepper to taste
- 3 ounces blue cheese crumbled
- ½ cup heavy whipping cream
- 1 small package frozen green beans

Directions:

1. Using your smallest burner, place a small pot over low heat, add a small amount of the heavy whipping cream and heat slightly before adding crumbled blue cheese. Melt the cheese stirring constantly. Once cheese is melted, raise heat slightly and stir in balance of whipping cream.
2. Continue cooking mixture on low until mixture reaches desired consistency. Turn heat off and move pot slightly off the burner and let it sit there until pork chops are ready to eat.
3. Heat a medium skillet to medium heat and add 2 tablespoons butter or olive oil. Add pork chops to hot pan and brown cooking approximately 2 minutes, depending on thickness of meat. Flip the meat to brown opposite side for another 2 minutes. Add salt and pepper to taste.
4. Microwave frozen green beans and season to taste.
5. Using two large plates, add a pork chop to each and divide blue cheese sauce and drizzle over pork chops.
6. Place green beans on plate and serve.

Week 4 Final Phase 2 **Finish Line** **Saturday** Breakfast

Baked Egg with Canadian Bacon and Tomato

Serves One

Ingredients:

- Butter or olive oil to coat ramekin
- 1 slice Canadian bacon
- 1 thin slice tomato
- 1 egg
- Salt and pepper to taste

Directions:

1. Heat oven to 375 degrees
2. Coat a ramekin with butter or olive oil
3. Line ramekin with Canadian bacon
4. Add a thin slice tomato on top of bacon
5. Break egg into ramakin and sprinkle with cheese of your choice.
6. Sit ramekin on oven tray and place in oven to bake.
7. Bake for approximately 10 minute or until desired doneness.
8. Add salt and pepper to taste.

Note: You are free to make two ramekin servings if you choose.

"The secret of health for both mind and body is not to mourn for the past, worry about the future, or anticipate troubles, but to live in the present moment wisely and earnestly."

— Buddha

Week 4 Final Phase 2 **Finish Line** **Saturday** Lunch

Zucchini Pizza

Serves Two

Ingredients:

- 2 medium zucchinis
- 1 tablespoon olive oil
- Himalayan Pink Salt
- Ground black pepper
- ½ cup Rau's Pizza Sauce
- ¾ cup shredded mozzarella
- ¼ cup grated Parmesan, plus extra for garnish
- ½ teaspoon oregano
- ¼ teaspoon basil
- 1/3 cup pepperoni

Directions:

1. Preheat oven to 450 degrees.
2. Cut zucchini lengthwise and scoop out centers and set aside, leaving just the shells.
3. Place 4 shells in a 9 x 9-inch or 7 x 11-inch baking pan
4. Chop up the reserved zucchini centers until very small and place in a medium sized bowl. Add salt, pepper, oregano, basil, pizza sauce, ½ cup mozzarella and Parmesan to the bowl and stir mixture until well blended.
5. Scoop mixture evenly into zucchini shells. Spread pepperoni slices on top of shells and divide remaining mozzarella between the four shells.
6. Place Zucchini Pizza in oven for approximate 20 minutes or until nicely browned.
7. Garnish with grated Parmesan cheese and serve.

Week 4 Final Phase 2 **Finish Line** **Saturday** Dinner

Baked Tilapia and Lemon Butter with Sweet Potato

Serves Two

Ingredients:

Note: Preheat oven to 400 degrees for sweet potatoes, and bake them before you prepare fish.

- 2 tilapia filets, you may use salmon if you choose
- Himalayan Pink Salt
- Freshly Ground Black Pepper
- 2 tablespoon butter
- 1 clove garlic, crushed
- Pinch red pepper flakes, optional
- ½ lemon sliced into thin rounds

Directions:

1. Choose a large skillet and melt butter on medium heat.
2. Add crushed garlic to skillet and sauté until tender. Add tilapia to skillet skin side up and cook for one minute. Carefully flip fish over and sprinkle with pepper flakes, and using other half of lemon, squeeze desired amount on fish. Add lemon rounds on and around fish.
3. Tilapia cooks very quickly so be careful not to overcook this delicate fish.
4. Remove fish to plates add salt and pepper to taste.

SweetPotato

Ingredients:

- 2 small sweet potatoes
- 4 tablespoons butter
- Salt and pepper to taste

Directions:

1. Preheat oven to 400 degrees
2. Scrub potatoes and wrap in foil
3. Place on oven rack in hot oven if well sealed or small baking pan for 40 to 45 minutes, depending on size of potato.
4. Using a pot holder, gently squeeze potato to test doneness.
5. Remove from oven and place one on each plate. You may slice the foil with a knife and squeeze potato open or carefully remove foil and cut potato open.
6. Add butter and any seasoning you choose.

Week 4 Final Phase 2 **Finish Line** **Sunday** Breakfast

Greek Omelet with Spinach and Feta Cheese

Serves Two

Ingredients:

- 1 bag organic baby spinach
- 4 large eggs
- 2 tablespoons olive oil
- 1 tablespoon butter
- Himalayan Pink Salt to taste
- Black pepper to taste

Directions:

1. Add olive oil to medium skillet and heat to medium. Add spinach and sauté. Remove spinach from pan and set aside to cool.
2. Place eggs in medium bowl and whisk. Add salt, pepper, spinach and feta cheese to eggs and whisk.
3. Reheat skillet and add butter to any olive oil left in skillet. Place egg mixture in skillet and stir until eggs mixture is fully cooked.
4. Serve with Keto Puff Bread

"The future is not a result of choices among alternative paths offered by the present, but a place that is created—created first in the mind and will, created next in activity. The future is not some place we are going to, but one we are creating. The paths are not to be found, but made, and the activity of making them, changes both the maker and the destination."

— John Schaar, futurist

Week 4 Final Phase 2 **Finish Line** **Sunday** Lunch

Tuna Salad

Serves Two

Ingredients:

- 1 large can tuna, drained
- 1/3 cup mayonnaise
- 1 teaspoon Dijon mustard
- ¼ cup diced white onion
- 1 clove garlic, crushed
- 1 teaspoon parsley flakes
- 1 medium celery stalk, diced
- Himalayan Pink Salt and pepper to taste
- 3 cups mixed salad greens
- 1 Avocado peeled and sliced

Directions:

1. In a medium sized bowl, combine all ingredients except tuna and avocado. Stir until well combined and then mix in tuna.
2. Using two large plates or salad bowls, add 1 ½ cup salad greens to each and top with tuna mixture.
3. Divide avocado and place on top of tuna.

NOTE

One more dinner and I'm finished. Wow!

My thoughts:

How I feel:

I'm going to recommend Keto for Life to:

Starting Weight:

Weight Today:

Total Weight Loss:

Week 4 Final Phase 2 **Finish Line** **Sunday** Dinner

Italian Lasagna

Serves Eight

Ingredients for Noodle Layer:

- 3 large eggs
- 2 ½ cups riced cauliflower (riced cauliflower now comes in frozen bags)
- 1 cup shredded mozzarella cheese
- Himalayan Pink Salt

Ingredients for Meat Filling:

- 1 tablespoon olive oil
- 1-pound ground beef
- 1 teaspoon Italian seasoning
- Himalayan Pink Salt
- Ground black pepper to taste
- 1 cup Rau's Tomato Sauce

Ingredients for Cheese Filling:

- 1 cup ricotta cheese
- 8 ounces shredded mozzarella, divided
- ¼ cup grated Parmesan
- 1 large egg, beaten
- 1 teaspoon Italian seasoning
- Himalayan Pink Salt
- Ground black pepper
- Chopped fresh parsley, for garnish

Directions:

1. Preheat oven to 350 degrees.
2. Line a large cookie sheet with parchment paper, making sure the paper lies flat so cauliflower mixture spreads out evenly.
3. Add eggs to a large bowl and beat, add cauliflower, 1 cup mozzarella, salt and mix together.
4. Pour mixture onto baking sheet, keeping it approximately ½ to ¾ inch thick.
5. Bake for 20 to 25 minutes until firm and golden being care-ful not to over brown or burn. Remove from oven and set aside to cool.
6. Increase oven temperature to 400 degrees.
7. Add olive oil and ground beef to a medium skillet and set on medium-high heat. Brown ground beef stirring constantly and breaking apart meat into small pieces. Do not overcook meat.
8. Add Rau's tomato sauce and cook mixture and stir for 2 minutes.
9. In a large bowl, beat 1 egg and add ricotta, ½ cup mozzarella, Parmesan cheese and Italian seasoning. Mix until combined. Add salt and pepper to taste.

Week 4 Final Phase 2 **Finish Line** **Sunday** Dinner

Italian Lasagna... cont. **Serves Two**

10. Coat an 8-inch x 8-inch baking pan with olive oil and add half of meat and cheese mixture to bottom of pan. Cut the cooled cauliflower layer into 2-inch-wide strips and add to baking sheet over layer of beef mixture. Add remaining meat mixture and balance of cauliflower noodles. Top mixture with ¼ cup shredded mozzarella.
11. Place in hot oven and bake for 20 minutes, until heated through and golden brown.

I sincerely hope you will continue to make Keto for Life your forever lifestyle eating plan. We have so much more knowledge available to us today, and the research is there at the click of a mouse. Be your own health advocate and always remember that we have made fad dieting a thing of the past. We have replaced it with Keto for Life!

— Barbara

Keto for Life Recipe Index

Breakfast Recipes / Week 1 Jumpstart

Breakfast Recipes / Week 2 Jumpstart

Breakfast Recipes / Week Three Phase 2 Push

Breakfast Recipes / Final Phase Victory

Lunch Recipes / Week 1 Jumpstart

Lunch Recipes / Week 2 Jumpstart

Lunch Recipes / Week 3 Phase 2 Push

Lunch Recipes / Week 4 Final Phase Victory

Dinner Recipes / Week 1 Jumpstart

Dinner Recipes / Week 2 Jumpstart

Dinner Recipes / Week 3 Phase 2 Push

Dinner Recipes / Week 4 Final Phase Victory

CITED WORKS

Chapter 1

1. *Keto Clarity: Your Definitive Guide to the Benefits of a Low-Carb, High-Fat Diet* by Jimmy Moore and Eric Westman M.D., Victory Bell Publishing, Inc., 2014.

2. *Grain Brain, The Surprising Truth About Wheat, Carbs, and Sugar—Your Brain's Silent Killers,* by David Perlmutter, M.D. 2013.

3. *Wheat Belly, Lose the Wheat Lose the Weight, and Find Your Path Back to Health,* by William Davis, MD 2011.

4. ***www.mercola.com,*** Health and Wellness Website, by Dr. Joseph Mercola

5. The Brain Maker, the Power of Gut Microbes to Heal and Protect Your Brain—for Life, by David Perlmutter, MD 2015.

6. Steven Nissen, chairman of the department of cardiovascular medicine at the Cleveland Clinic.

7. Article by Anahad O'Connor for The New York Times on September 1, 2014

Chapter 2

1. *The Great Cholesterol Myth, Why Lowering Your Cholesterol Won't Prevent Heart Disease and the Statin-Free Plan that Will,* by Jonny Bowden, PH.D., C.N.S. and Stephen Sinatra, MD., F.A.C.C., Fair Winds Press 2012.

2. *Dr. Atkin's New Diet Revolution,* by Robert C. Atkin's MD, HarperCollins Publishers, 2002.

3. *Always Hungry, Conquer Cravings, Retrain Your Fat Cells & Lose Weight Permanently,* Dr. Ludwig, MD, Ph.D., Grand Central Publishing, 2016.

4. According to Anne Alexander, Editorial Director of Prevention, "The average American consumes 130 pounds of added sugar per year—that is, sugar that's an ingredient in food rather than sugar that is naturally occurring in food," by Anne Alexander, Editorial Director of Prevention 2016.

Chapter 3

1. Research provided by the Journal of the Academy of Nutrition and Diabetes, they concluded that 73 percent of packaged foods purchased in grocery stores contain added sugars.

2. Harvard Magazine article titled, *Are all Calories Equal?* June 2016.

3. According to psychology professor Bart Hoebel, who specializes in the neuroscience of appetite, weight and sugar addiction, "Some people have

claimed that high-fructose corn syrup is no different than other sweeteners when it comes to weight gain and obesity."

4. A major study conducted by Princeton University comparing weight gain and high-fructose corn syrup

5. *That Sugar Film,* a documentary produced by filmmaker Damon Gameau, study showed the health effects of a high sugar diet on a healthy body.

6. Robert H. Lustig, M.D., M.S.I., *Fat Chance, Beating the Odds Against Sugar, Processed Food, Obesity, and Disease.*

7. SugarScience.org, study shows sugar is added to 74 percent of processed foods and it is disguised under 60 different names.

8. Study from the National Academy of Sciences USA, using fMRI imaging scans on 24 volunteers to test their brain reaction to fructose versus glucose.

9. A postdoctoral fellow at U.C.S.F., Cristin E. Kerns, exposed documents discovered in 1964 in the archives at Harvard. The papers, purposed a plan to influence public opinion on the safety of sugar.

10. *The Urban Monk, Eastern Wisdom and Modern Hacks to Stop Time and Find Success, Happiness and Peace,* by Pedram Shojai, OMD, published by Rodale Inc., 2016.

Chapter 4

1. *Nutrition Watchdog,* Mike Geary, Certified Nutrition Specialist and bestselling author, says AGE's or Advanced Glycation End Products, actually speed up aging in your body. Wheat is the culprit.

2. Dr. David Perlmutter, author of *Brain Maker.*

3. New York Times article by Jane E. Brody, on November 16, 2017, paints a dark picture of the dangers of weight gain.

4. *Wheat Belly Cookbook, 150 Recipes to Lose the Weight, and Find Your Path Back to Health,* by William Davis MD, Rodale, 2013.

5. *The Framingham Heart Study,* researcher Dr. George Mann, 1948-1968.

6. *Life Line Screening,* article on belly fat by Joelle Reizer, March 10, 2015.

7. *The Rosedale Diet, Turn off Your Hunger Switch, Live Longer, Lose Weight Fast, and Keep It Off,* by Ron Rosedale, MD, and Carol Coleman, HarperCollins, 2004.

Chapter 5

1. The American Heart Association (AHA) and the National Heart, Lung and Blood Institute (NHLBI) on metabolic syndrome.

2. An article in the *New York Times* titled Obesity and Diabetes Tied to Liver Cancer, *New York Times,* October 14, 2016, by Nicholas Bakalar.

3. Dr. Eric Westman from his book *Keto Clarity.*

4. National Heart, Lung, and Blood Institute.

5. *Your Personal Paleo Code, Eat Right for Your Genes, Body Type, and Personal Health Needs—Prevent and Reverse Disease, Lose Weight Effortlessly and look and Feel Better than Ever,* by Chris Kresser, an alternative medicine teacher, 2014.

6. Dr. Stephen Guyenet, obesity researcher on the science of body and weight.

Chapter 7

1. The Telomere Effect, A Revolutionary Approach to Living Younger, Healthier, Longer.

2. February 2017 *Harvard Health Letter,* titled "What can you do to avoid Alzheimer's disease?"

3. AARP from the Stanford Center on Longevity by Laura L. Christensen; it stated that cognitive decline is not inevitable.

4. John Medina, affiliate professor of bioengineering at the University of Washington School of Medicine and author of *Brain Rules.*

Chapter 8

1. A study by researchers at Rush University Medical Center in Chicago, Illinois on goals and purpose.

Chapter 9

1. A study reported in January 2013 by *The Journal of Nutrition and Cancer,* revealed the power of photo chemicals found in avocados can aid in cancer cell death.

2. January 2013 by *The Journal of Nutrition and Cancer,* revealed the power of photochemical found in avocados.

3. According to studies in the *American Journal of Clinical Nutrition,* risk of type 2 diabetes may be lower in daily consumption of cheese.

4. Dr. William J. Blot of National Cancer Institute reported on large studies of people in China and Italy on benefits of garlic.

5. A study by researchers at Columbia University Medical Center in New York, on 2000 on the Mediterranean diet.

6. A study done in 1996 and posted in the journal *Cancer, Epidemiology, Biomarkers & Prevention,* stated that consuming cruciferous vegetables lowered risk of cancer.

7. A study at Rush University Medical Center showed that leafy greens have an anti-aging effect due to vitamin K, folate, lutein, and beta-carotene presence.

Barbara's Weight Loss Group Coaching Program

If you are struggling to get the weight off, and more importantly keep it off, consider joining my weight loss group coaching program. Learn how the Ketogentic Diet combats inflammation in the body and puts you on the path to wellness.

Unfortunately, many still hang on to the old paradigm that "a calorie is a calorie," or "fat makes you fat," and you need "sugar for energy."

This is simply not true! The body is not satiated when consuming low fat and fat-free fake food, which causes massive weight gain—as is obvious from our expanding waistlines.

Together we will explore ways to provide an understanding of how emotions play into overeating and how to recognize ways we sabotage our weight loss plan.

Barbara's Weight Loss Group Coaching Program is a perfect place to start on the path to wellness. The group will hold you accountable, but more importantly, provide the support and encouragement to keep you on track to your weight loss goal.

Contact Barbara today!

Barbara@BarbaraAndCompany.com

https://www.BarbaraAndCompany.com

About Barbara

For the last 20 years, Barbara Miller has made it a life mission to bring awareness to the causes of expanding waistlines, heart disease and diabetes. After the painful loss of her mother to heart disease, she began passionately studying and researching health and wellness and the dangers of a high carbohydrate diet. Watching the obesity epidemic surge in recent years was a major factor in writing this book. Barbara believes awareness is critical to protecting the only body you will ever have, and one of the best ways to do this is through the food you eat! As a health and wellness entrepreneur, she believes diet and exercise are the two deciding factors to a quality life that everyone so richly deserves.

Barbara Miller, author, motivational speaker, and certified master life coach is the founder of Barbara & Company International Inc. Barbara studied Health and Wellness at Ashford University, and also studied at Kendall College of Art & Design. She earned her master life coaching certification through American University of NLP, and health coach certification through Evercoach: Health Coaching, Cynthia Garcia.

You can reach Barbara at: Barbara@BarbaraAndCompany.com

www.BarbaraAndCompany.com www.KetoForLifeBlog.com

I sincerely want to thank you for purchasing and reading this book. It is my deepest desire that you find the answers you are searching for in the pages of *Keto for Life.*

Please visit my new blog and click the 'like' button at: www.KetoForLifeblog.com where I will be posting valuable tips and information, plus videos, and new recipes. You may post and leave comments, as well as ask questions on the blog.

Please go to my FaceBook author page and click the 'like' button at:
www.facebook.com/BarbaraMillerAuthor

Please visit my Twitter page and click the 'follow' button and write a tweet at:
www.twitter.com/BarbaraSMiller

Please visit my Pinterest page and follow my boards at:
www.pinterest.com/BarbaraMAuthor/pins/

Please visit my website and opt-in for my monthly newsletter at:
www.BarbaraAndCompany.com

Follow me on Instagram: https://instagram.com/BarbaraSueMiller

— Barbara Miller

CPSIA information can be obtained
at www.ICGtesting.com
Printed in the USA
LVHW012140071019
633403LV00009B/3359/P